YOGI BARE

*Naked Truth from
America's Leading Yoga Teachers*

PHILIP SELF

Cypress Moon Press
NASHVILLE, TENNESSEE

Cypress Moon Press
P.O. Box 210925
Nashville, TN 37221
cypmoon@aol.com

The following grateful acknowledgments are made for permission to reprint excerpts from previously published material:

"Mrs. Rosemary" in SEE ROCK CITY by Donald Davis (August House, 1996). Copyright 1996 by Donald Davis, Storyteller, Inc. Reprinted by permission.

TURN! TURN! TURN!
(To Everything There Is a Season)
Words from the Book of Ecclesiastes
Adaptation and Music by Pete Seeger
TRO –©– Copyright 1962 (Renewed) Melody Trails, Inc., New York, NY
Used by Permission

Self, Philip, 1960-
    Yogi bare : naked truth from America's leading yoga
Teachers / Philip Self. — 1st ed.
    p.   cm.
    Includes bibliographical references.
    ISBN: 0-9666894-0-2

    1. Yogis — Spiritual life — Interviews.   2. Yoga.
I. Title

BL1171.S45 1998   294.5'0922
                                         QBI98-1228

First Cypress Moon Press trade paperback printing September 1998

10 9 8 7 6 5 4 3 2

Cover photo of Richard Freeman in *urdhva kukkutasana* by Jonathan Pite.

Typography and design by Roger A. DeLiso, Nashville, Tennessee.

Printed in the United States of America

YOGI BARE

To Bryan,
the best guru a father could have

I am only acting as a mirror for your life,
in which you can see yourself as you are;
then you can throw away the mirror;
the mirror is not important.

—J. KRISHNAMURTI

TABLE OF CONTENTS

INTRODUCTION

The alarm clock shook me at 4:30 a.m., rudely awakening me to the life of an author. I had flown into New York City's La Guardia Airport the night before. After a harrowing cab ride and a $25.00 late-night midtown breakfast where dry toast cost more than the $2.50 cup of coffee, I finally climbed into bed at 1:30 in the morning.

I fumbled in the dark to stop the obnoxious buzzing. I stumbled to the bathroom, flipped on what could have passed for an interrogation lamp, and splashed water on my aching face as I tried to shake the cobwebs out of my brain that was begging, along with my body, for more sleep. I took a quick first shower, threw on some clothes, ate a day-old muffin, and grabbed my backpack, which contained a note pad, three pens, two cassette recorders, extra batteries, a towel, and a change of clothes.

My bloodshot eyes could have been used as a map for the railways of Amtrak, which was where I had to be in one hour to catch the 79 at 6:15 to Philadelphia. Baron Baptiste was meeting me at the 30th Street Station, and I was to attend a morning class at his Power Yoga Institute in Bryn Mawr, Pennsylvania. I had taken a class with Baron at the *Yoga Journal* Conference in San Francisco a month earlier, so I was prepared to sweat. After a much-needed second shower, I would conduct my first interview for *Yogi Bare* with Baron over lunch.

I arrived at Penn Station after a less harrowing cab ride than the night before. (Not a lot of city folk up at 5:30 a.m., and those who are haven't been to bed.) I handed the conductor my ticket, and I was on my way to Philly. Although my eyes wanted to close, I resisted the temptation. If I fell asleep during the ninety-minute train ride, I would be in serious danger of waking up in a puddle of drool to the sound of "Next stop Washington, D.C." I wasn't sure if the President practiced yoga, but I was fairly certain I would not be able to score an interview with him on such short notice.

The interview with Baron was a close call. He was leaving with his family for Hawaii the following day, and I didn't know when I would be back on the East Coast. His generosity of juggling a busy schedule was the first of many similar scenarios of selflessness I encountered in the course of writing this book. According to Martin Pierce, "Yoga helps people to be more truly caring towards others." (Incidentally, Martin, who was traveling to New England with his daughters the day after our interview, juggled his schedule as well.) I have found that selflessness is how you find your Self.

I managed to stay awake, get off the train, and meet Baron. As we drove to his studio and I told him more about myself and the project, we passed a man walking down the street who bore a striking resemblance to Michael Gliksohn, then publisher of the *Yoga Journal*. We did a double take, laughed, and I knew life was giving me confirmation, albeit through a preposterous and improbable sign, that I was headed down the right road.

ॐ

The idea for *Yogi Bare* was born one week before the 2nd Annual *Yoga Journal* Conference, which I had no intention of attending. However, that particular evening after practicing yoga and meditation, my inner voice prompted me to attend the conference and write an interview book with America's leading yoga teachers.

"But it's one week before the conference!" my logical mind objected.

Nevertheless, I picked up a back issue of the *Yoga Journal* and opened it at random to the ad for the conference. What more confirmation does one need? Although I had never met Erich Schiffmann, I took the advice he would later dispense in an interview: "Dare to do as you are prompted to do." The next morning, I booked a flight, booked a room, and began a book.

I knew four teachers who were presenting at the conference. I had attended weekend workshops with Rodney Yee and Thom and Beryl Bender Birch in Nashville. And I had taken a number of classes with Rod Stryker over the course of a year while on business trips to the West Coast. I shared with each of them my meditation-driven book idea. Incredibly, they all agreed to be interviewed by an unknown writer who had never written a book. That's faith. Over the next nine months, I conducted twenty face-to-face interviews all across the country with America's leading yoga teachers. That's grace.

I began practicing yoga three years prior to the *Yoga Journal* conference, because I intuitively believed it would help with lower back problems I was experiencing. I went to a local video store and found three yoga tapes available—two by celebrities and one by Patricia Walden, a teacher I had never heard of. Even though I work in the entertainment industry, I bypassed the celebrity fare in favor of *Yoga Journal's Practice for Beginners*. Thus, Patricia became my first yoga teacher via video.

The second day of the conference, I saw Patricia Walden at lunch. I recognized her from the video the same way someone might recognize a rock star, although to my knowledge, Patricia has never been on MTV. (However, Baron Baptiste is working on a project for MTV Japan.) I went over, introduced myself, and thanked her for giving me the gift of yoga. Of course, I wanted to ask her to be in the book, but the moment didn't feel right. Maybe I was following the advice of my literary guru, Mark Twain: "Do not offer a compliment and ask for a favor at the same time. A compliment that is charged for is not valuable." (Ever notice that Lahiri Mahasaya looks like Samuel Clemens sans cigar?)

On the final day of the conference, I was sitting on my sticky mat meditating as I waited for the last class to begin. The room was packed with people who had signed up for a class with Baron. About a minute before class began, I heard someone roll out their sticky mat next to mine in the only available spot. When I opened my eyes and looked to my right, Patricia Walden was sitting beside me.

After the surreal experience of practicing yoga next to the contemporary teacher who introduced me to the ancient practice, I asked Patricia to participate in *Yogi Bare*. I found out later that we had both taken Baron's class on a lark. I believe the universe conspires for us and disguises it as coincidence. Or the quote Rama Berch shares: "Coincidence is God's way of remaining anonymous." Within a year following the conference, I serendipitously ran into Patricia in New York City and Los Angeles while on business trips.

One morning in early December, I began a three-hour drive from Nashville to Cincinnati for a two o'clock interview with Lilias Folan. When I told my wife I was interviewing Lilias, she said, "I used to do yoga with her on TV in the fifth grade." In fact, several teachers in *Yogi Bare* cite Lilias as an influence on their lives.

I allowed for a time zone change, time to eat lunch, and my

haplessly poor sense of direction. Although I am a white Anglo-Saxon Protestant, I am the direct opposite of a wasp. If you move a wasp's nest, the wasp will die trying to find it. The wasp can't find the nest, because he is absolutely certain where it is supposed to be. While a wasp seemingly bobs around haphazardly in flight, his sense of direction is superior to a swallow making a beeline to Capistrano. You don't even have to move my nest, and the odds are two-to-one I will drive right past it coming home from work. I've got neighbors standing on the corner every evening placing bets. Fortunately, the directions Lilias gave were impeccable and I arrived at 1:55. There is no such thing as being fashionable late to conduct an interview.

It was a wonderful day. I spent two-hours with Lilias, met her personable husband, Bob, did a little Christmas shopping, and hung around to take an evening yoga class. After class, Lilias and I said our good-byes and I headed back to Nashville.

I was no more than thirty minutes out of Cincinnati, when in my mind's eye, I saw my hand turning over the tape and my finger pushing play instead of record.

"Impossible!" my ego emphatically tried to reassure me. "You've done this eighteen times. You've flipped dozens of tapes without a hitch. You're just being paranoid."

"Can you be sure?" my doubt rebutted.

The simple thing would have been to listen to the tape, but since I had thrown my travel bag in the trunk before yoga class, it wasn't within reach. I didn't want to pull over on the emergency lane of I-75, as my dilemma didn't constitute a legitimate 911. For the next hour—no matter how many songs I sang along with—my mind raged the great debate of "did I, or didn't I?" I was more nerve-racked than a school girl with a crush and a daisy playing "he loves me, he loves me not." The difference was I couldn't simply pick another flower. And there's your trouble.

When I pulled into a Cracker Barrel (nothing but five-star restaurants for this author), I popped the trunk, fished out the tape recorder, put in the cassette tape with the alleged interview of Lilias Folan with the broken tabs to insure I wouldn't accidentally erase or record over it, rewound a few seconds, and pressed play.

Silence.

"Maybe you didn't rewind far enough," my hope encouraged.

I rewound a few more seconds and pressed play.

Silence.

Gone.

Side B of our interview was floating somewhere in the ether.

"Well, at least you recorded side A," my optimism consoled me.

Then I had one of those Stephen King thoughts that makes the heart race and the palms sweat. I vividly recalled after about two minutes into our interview, Lilias got a phone call. She excused herself to turn down the volume on the answering machine, so we wouldn't be disturbed. When she left the room, in an effort to conserve tape, I turned the recorder off. It suddenly occurred to me why the manufacturer puts a pause button on these gizmos.

As the shower scene music from *Psycho* danced in my head, my anxiety screamed, "WHAT IF YOU PUSHED PLAY INSTEAD OF RECORD WHEN SHE CAME BACK AND DIDN'T RECORD SIDE A EITHER!? WHAT IF YOU TOOK A VACATION DAY AND DROVE TO CINCINNATI AND BACK FOR NOTHING!?"

With fear and trepidation I rewound side A. The interview started. Yes! I listened with nail-biting anticipation for the next two minutes and heard the click where I turned the recorder off. I held my breath like a die-hard fan watching a last second "Hail Mary." I heard another clicking noise and the interview resumed. Touchdown!

I learned several things from that experience, more accurately termed a fiasco. First, things can always be worse. At least, I had side A on tape. And suppose I had not recorded side A. I could have taken solace in the fact that I didn't get a flat tire coming or going. Count your blessings.

Second, the mind's eye has 20/20 vision. My subconscious mind knew I pushed play instead of record. My conscious mind wanted to deny the truth. My subconscious wasn't trying to taunt me, merely inform me. I taunted myself. Trust your instincts.

Third, nothing is for nothing. Or as my favorite storyteller, Donald Davis, says through Mrs. Rosemary in his poignant and stirring tale of kindergarten, "Boys and girls, nothing ever dies for no reason. If something dies, it's either because it got too hurt to get well, or too sick to get well, or if it was really lucky, just plain too old to get well."

Finally, life's most valuable lessons must be learned first hand. As The Byrds sing:

> To everything turn, turn, turn
> There is a season turn, turn, turn
> And a time to every purpose under heaven

A time to record, a time to erase.

I have since learned that any recording engineer worth his salt has at least one horror story of when he went to red when he shouldn't have and erased thousands of dollars of recorded music, or forgot to push record and missed the take of a lifetime. We are never alone, even in our buffoonery.

When I tallied the day's ledger of debits and credits, it was a positive experience sans side B. I had been engaged in stimulating conversation, connected with a spiritual being posing as a human being, and practiced yoga. We tally our ledger with perception and attitude.

The irony in not recording side B of our interview is that on side A, Lilias speaks about mistakes. Particularly about how she had to learn to forgive herself for mistakes she made on the air. "If you are sensitive," Lilias divulges, "you think about people seeing this mistake time and time again." Thirty minutes later, I made an embarrassing mistake. I say it was embarrassing because there was no way of sweeping it under the rug. I had to reveal my error to Lilias, if I was to ever complete the interview. I hated making that call.

Lilias also said something else important about a mistake. She termed it a "miss take," which she asserted "you can do again and again until you get it right." I am here to report she stands behind her philosophy. One month later, after the hustle and bustle of Christmas and New Year's, we conducted a "re-take" of the "miss take" over the telephone. I loved making that call.

When compiling a list of people to interview for *Yogi Bare*, I attempted to present a cross section of the country, as well as different styles of yoga. I even included international voices of people who teach in America to broaden the scope. Unfortunately, it is impossible to represent every geographic region and every yogic tradition with twenty interviews. Nevertheless, it is a worthy representation of America's leading yoga teachers.

Picking twenty of America's leading yoga teachers is akin to picking an all-star team—some deserving person gets left off the roster. Case in point, the names of Judith Lasater and Joel Kramer kept cropping up. Working with the film industry, I understand the value of a sequel. Rocky Balboa has fought in more bouts than George Foreman. If there is a *Yogi Bare II*, I hope the above mentioned leading teachers will participate. However, I promise not to get carried away with the concept. If there is one more helping of *Chicken Soup for the Soul*, Jack Canfield and Mark Victor Hansen should be tarred-and-feathered. I'm on the verge of spiritual salmonella.

While I traveled extensively to obtain the interviews, several were conducted during weekend workshops in Nashville. You know the yoga community is well organized when we have snappy little buzzwords like "weekend workshop." They're fun. Sign up. You're worth it. Honor your practice.

When arranging the interviews, I listened to my inner voice. I suggest you do the same when deciding the order in which to read them. You may take my lead, or maybe you will decide to read the interviews from back to front. Maybe you will start with the odd-numbered interviews and then read the even-numbered. You could put twenty numbers in a hat, and draw and read until you are out of digits and chapters. Dealer's choice.

Writing this book has been a metamorphosis. The journey has shaped and molded me. Before I started *Yogi Bare*, I entertained romantic fantasies of idyllic travel to India. Now after hearing numerous tales of hepatitis, chaotic travel, and near-death experiences, the Himalayas are not in my immediate travel plans. At the present moment, I'll opt for *National Geographic Explorer*. Give me a leather chair, a roaring fire, and *India Unveiled* by Robert Arnett. I'll take a vicarious adventure with Anne Cushman and Jerry Jones' *From Here to Nirvana: Yoga Journal's Guide to Spiritual India*. Nevertheless, I must admit John Friend weaves a fascinating and entertaining tale of his travels to the seat of yoga by the seat of his pants.

The journey has also empowered me. Any time you complete a project, especially one of passion, you evolve. If I said bringing this vision to fruition was easy, I would be lying. I wrote *Yogi Bare* while working a full-time job and serving a life-term as husband and father. For those scoring at home, that's a life-term as in Supreme

Court justice, not prisoner.

The ultimate irony is that the time, commitment, discipline, and energy required for writing a book on yoga teachers encroached upon my yoga practice. I often reminded myself of the words of Richard Freeman: "Staying balanced requires you to see all things as sacred, because occasionally you will miss your practice."

If I can impart one thing I learned along the way, it would be this—listen to your inner voice and follow your heart.

As Gabriella Giubilaro related, "My heart was telling me to teach yoga and my brain was telling me to stay at the university. One day, I told myself if I don't run the risk and try to teach yoga, later in life I would regret it. If I couldn't teach yoga, at least I would know I tried. I thought it was important to follow my heart."

Follow your heart.

When I moved to Nashville to break into the music business, I kept my head above water by being a food consultant specializing in retail sales. One day, the restaurant manager, Bill Nagel, said something at a staff meeting that I will never forget: "If you do something half-ass, then you are half-ass." I have done my best to make *Yogi Bare* full-ass. (Or should that be ass-less?) Anyway, you get the point. If you are going to go to the trouble of doing something, do your best to do it right.

My mother adheres to this philosophy. When I was growing up and halfheartedly doing chores, she would follow behind me with the white glove. After re-washing windows, re-dusting furniture, and re-vacuuming carpet, I soon learned it was easier and quicker to do something right the first time. I am grateful for this discipline training. While I always try to work smarter, there is no substitute for hard work. If nothing else, I hope you will read my effort between the lines.

Bill Nagel, now a successful personal fitness trainer, left the restaurant to open an aerobics and fitness center called Power Source. He was a visionary and ahead of his time. Power Source offered yoga. You couldn't say that about too many fitness centers in the mid-eighties. Now it's commonplace. The wave of yoga that started in the sixties has moved into the mainstream.

A few of us from the restaurant decided to take a yoga class and support Bill. I didn't want to walk into Power Source totally ignorant, so just like some of the yogis in this book, I went out and bought a yoga book by Richard Hittleman. I flipped through the pages and proclaimed, "I can do this. Piece of cake." So as a young man in my mid-twenties and full of arrogance, I headed off to yoga class.

The aerobics teacher who had dabbled in yoga proceeded to lead the class through ninety minutes of rigorous stretching. Not only was I doing what Joel Kramer calls "playing the edge," I was over the edge. I was competing with the class for "Most Flexible Virgo."

I wish Bryan Kest had been around to warn me—"We love to compete, but competition hinders our practice." The next morning, I needed a block and tackle to get out of bed.

It would be ten years before I ventured near *trikonasana* again.

Fortunately, I found a great teacher in Patricia Walden the second time around. I bought the *Yoga Journal's Practice for Beginners*, brought it home, and popped it in my VCR. As I watched Patricia perform her five-minute demonstration in Death Valley, I was immediately inspired and intimidated. My spirit had been seduced, and my physical body was about to be molded into various postures my mind had never conceived. Little did I know my subtle body would be molded as well.

My diet began to change. I am not alone in this phenomenon. As Rodney Yee shares, "When I started doing my *asana* practice, the postures started cleansing me to the point where I didn't desire meat. It wasn't something that I had to discipline myself to become. Becoming a vegetarian happened organically." Gabriella Giubilaro echoes Rodney's sentiment: "I became vegetarian three years after I started to do yoga—and not out of decision. It came by itself."

Although, I am not one-hundred-percent vegetarian, the organic changes in my dietary habits have been significant. Having grown up in the South, I was used to consuming meat three meals a day with a snack of beef jerky or pork rinds thrown in for good measure. Now I partake of tofu on a regular basis.

Also, my self-perception would change. Speaking on *asana* Patricia Walden relates, "You would think that would stop at the physical plane, but it seeps into many layers of your being. You start to feel differently about yourself, and then people start responding to you differently. I see so clearly in my students how the practice of *asana* builds self-esteem and makes them feel adequate." Amen, Sister! Amen!

If you practice yoga, or aspire to do so, find a great teacher. If you are a yoga teacher, conduct a great class. A great class is a class that's appropriate for the student. The teacher and the student should both employ this wisdom.

The issue of national teaching standards is currently being debated amongst the yoga community. Eighteen countries comprising the European Union of Yoga have adopted teaching standards. Rama Berch, who terms the debate "the yoga of the yoga teachers," states, "It's an important issue because yoga is becoming such a strong river of consciousness. I have lived with that question for over two years, and I have been on both sides of it—yea and nay."

Sandra Summerfield Kozak adds, "The practice of yoga creates more comfort on all levels in people's lives. But yoga can only be that resource if taught by educated teachers who themselves understand what yoga is."

Rod Stryker offers, "I was taught that the teacher should be careful of who he picks as a student. The student should be as careful as the teacher is. You should only have faith in the teacher to the degree in which your work with him verifies your trust."

Though currently in favor of national teaching standards, Rama concludes, "Yoga traditionally has not been about external standards at all. If the teacher is bad, people quit going to them."

The aerobics teacher at Power Source should have asked if anyone was new to yoga. She should have introduced herself to the "new faces" and inquired about their yoga practice, if any. And I should have informed her that I had never done yoga before. Take responsibility for your yoga.

More than once I have pondered where my practice would be today if yoga had resonated that fateful day we first met many years ago in an aerobics studio. But I have come to accept that things stick when we are ready for them. As Julie Lawrence shares, "Yoga has taught me that everything happens in its own time." When yoga came around the second time, I was ready. I have stuck with the sticky mat ever since.

I am fortunate to have had the privilege of being initiated by some of the best yogis America has to offer. Patricia Walden introduced me to Iyengar yoga. I ventured back to the video store after a month of practice with Patricia's beginners tape and purchased Rodney Yee's *Yoga Journal's Practice for Strength*. I later attended my first weekend workshop with Rodney. Desiring to know more about various yoga styles, I was introduced to *ashtanga* yoga by Thom and

Beryl Bender Birch. I attended my first yoga retreat with Erich Schiffmann. Gary Kraftsow introduced me to *Viniyoga*. Unfortunately, it wasn't on Maui.

A tropical storm heading towards Martha's Vineyard kept me in New York City longer than I anticipated. That weekend, Alan Finger introduced me to meditation. Alan also referred me to Rod Stryker, with whom I had my first private. Los Angeles is a fairly large place. When I first met Rod, he was teaching a mere fifteen blocks from my hotel. If you have ever driven on the 101 during rush hour traffic, you know that is not only miraculous, it's a godsend.

I first experienced Sanskrit with Vyaas Houston. Although I enjoyed chanting, I must admit foreign language has never been my forte. After twelve hours of German at Louisiana Tech University, I am hard pressed to count to ten in Deutsche without the benefit of at least *ein* stein of pilsner.

Each of the above mentioned yogis, along with the other participants of *Yogi Bare*, are shaping the future of Western yoga. After reading these interviews, I think you will agree we're in good hands.

When I began *Yogi Bare*, I had no idea what an important role the Internet would play. I e-mailed files, corresponded to other continents, and checked out the web pages of Gabriel Halpern, Bryan Kest, Gary Kraftsow, and Erich Schiffmann. I even located Robert Wisehart to compile the glossary.

You may be asking, "Why didn't you compile it yourself?"

Answer: Because I am not a Sanskrit scholar. Or in Nagelese: "If you do something half-ass, then you are half-ass."

"But you interviewed Vyaas Houston, a Sanskrit scholar. Why didn't you employ his services?"

I thought of that one, Jagadis Chandra Bose. I was born at

night, but not last night. Unfortunately, Vyaas was in the midst of teaching summer Sanskrit intensives.

"What to do?" my perseverance inquired.

After a couple of cold trails, I went to the World Wide Web and typed "Sanskrit" into a search engine. If I had been guessing "high/low" on how many Sanskrit web sites there are on the *Price is Right*, Bob Barker would have definitely said, "Higher."

In less than one hour, I had located Robert Wisehart and had spoken to him by telephone halfway across this great land. I ended up with a quality glossary and a new friend. Trust the universe.

When I was a student at Candler School of Theology at Emory University, one of my professors said, "We can never know the answers; we can only hope to ask better questions." This seemed a peculiar environment to hear such a comment, since religion is hell-bent on definitive answers.

Maybe it was the irony of the venue that caused his comment to remain with me through the years as I have attempted to ask better questions and let go of my attachment to the answers. If I know the answer, what is the point of the question?

As Donna Farhi eloquently stated, "Practicing yoga doesn't mean you answer your questions. It means you learn to live with your questions, rather than having some kind of righteousness that you have answered them. You remain open-minded all the time, because there may be another possibility you haven't considered."

Maybe I could have asked better questions in the interviews, but there is no shortage of wisdom between the pages of *Yogi Bare*. Let the wisdom of the answers remind you that your truest answers lie within, if you dare to ask the questions.

Over the years, the two best questions I have asked, although admittedly unoriginal, are "Who am I?" and "What do I need to know?" I ask these daily. One time my inner voice replied, "Who said that?" and "Beats me." Sometimes I am humbled by the response and must modify my behavior. Sometimes I am challenged to my highest potential. Every time I sit with these two questions in meditation, there is something new to discover from the universal fountain of truth.

Establish a meditation practice.

Life cannot be described; it can only be experienced.

As Rama Berch imparts, "If you have never eaten a chocolate-covered strawberry, anything I try to tell you about that experience is going to be incomplete. How do you tell someone what it's like? You give them a chocolate-covered strawberry and they go, 'Ah.'"

Accordingly, it is impossible to recreate the magic of each interview in *Yogi Bare*. You really had to be there. On several occasions, I conducted an interview with an interested silent observer present. They can vouch for me.

The interview process is organic. While there is definite preparation and you have a general direction in mind, you must be willing to trust the flow of the current. The interview is as likely to change course as the Ganges River, as it twists and turns on its way to the Bay of Bengal. "You're letting the flow flow," Erich Schiffmann enlightens.

I am amazed at the honesty with which people shared their lives—especially the difficult and trying times. But that is one of the measures of a great teacher.

"Yoga teachers are not perfect beings, although students like to think of us as such," Lilias Folan confides. "It's just not true."

I would choose a teacher who is honest over a teacher who is perfect, if such a thing existed.

Students are not perfect either, but we shouldn't lament. John Friend proposes quite the opposite: "You are supreme, and there is tremendous goodness and worthiness inside of you. Find the blessing in your limitations, instead of seeing them as a curse."

While each teacher gives insight into their story, the objective is for them to give you insight into your own story. As Gabriel Halpern comments, "You can listen to the story of someone else's life to get a clue, but then you have to carom off that and listen to your own heart." Their trials and tribulations, and triumphs and celebrations should remind you of the sacredness of your journey and inspire you to reflect upon your life. You have to know where you came from to know where you're going. And between the two lives the present moment.

J. Krishnamurti said, "I am only acting as a mirror for your life, in which you can see yourself as you are; then you can throw away the mirror; the mirror is not important."

I hope you don't throw *Yogi Bare* away. And I hope this book doubles as a mirror.

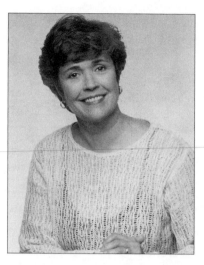

LILIAS FOLAN

CINCINNATI

You introduced millions of people to yoga through your nationally syndicated PBS television shows Lilias! *and* Lilias, Yoga and You. *How does it feel to be the Grand Dame of American Yoga?*

I love it and I feel very honored. It is exciting every time I hear people's PBS television yoga stories. It's amazing how something that began in 1972 had an influence and continues to influence millions of people all over the United States. At the time, I had absolutely no idea it would have such an impact. I know I could not have done anything else with my life. Television is a part of my being. I am so grateful I had the opportunity. People ask me, "Did you think about it when you started?" My answer is what Krishnamurti said, "If the house is burning you get up and put out the fire."

That's really what it felt like—there was a house burning, and I had to get up and put out the fire.

What was the inspiration for Lilias, Yoga and You?

I had the bee in my bonnet that I wanted to do a television series, and, certainly, I was inspired by Richard Hittleman's yoga show. I thought, "I'm learning something from this man, but I can do this better." I also liked how Julia Child communicated through the glass. Those two shows were always pushing me to have my own show.

I have a dramatic family. My great-grandfather, Reuben Osborne Moon, was a fine orator in the Senate. My mother is a fine speaker. My brother has been an actor, and now he's a filmmaker. They gave me the inspiration to say, "I can do this. I've never been trained, but by golly, I'm going to learn how to communicate clearly, to speak up, and remember that diction is important."

You have to be able to express yourself to a television camera when nobody is there except two cameramen who are very bored. You don't have a class of a hundred interested people sitting in front of you. It's a very different energy. Taylor Feltnor, my director who has worked with me producing the *Lilias!* series for PBS for many years, said, "I know more about yoga than I *ever* wanted to know!"

I taped over five hundred classes. The last fifty-two were the ones where I began to mature. Sitting in front of and working with a camera, I got the inner message, "Say what you want to say, because you might not get another opportunity to do this." I really worked hard at taking it seriously, digging deep, and going to my edges as far as what I wanted to say to an American who had never thought about yoga, or to someone who thought it was crazy and off the wall. I wanted to make it as reachable and as American as possible.

What did you want to say about yoga?

I have never had a plan. I just wanted to try to be myself. I wanted to communicate the essence of yoga is one's own divinity, but I could never come out and say, point blank, "Find out who you are. Ask yourself the most important question of your life, 'Who am I?'"

I learned that if you share who *you* are with people, it will naturally help them reflect on who they are. A lot of the television show was sharing my own experience, but the postures, the breathing, and the relaxation was woven through it. The underlying message was, "Know thyself," and the importance of universal love. If you are loving with no strings attached, even through the medium of television, people can feel it. I have had countless letters from people saying, "I can feel your caring." Human beings will bloom if you come from that place inside yourself. You don't have to say anything, but if you come from the core of universal love, everything else will follow. It has taken years for me to understand that.

It sounds like the key was being sincere and authentic.

Yes. Being sincere, authentic, and as real as I could possibly be. You put powder and paint on your face, and you care about what color leotards you wear. Being on camera and having people look at you brings a false sense of reality. I had to always deal with that inside of myself. I came to understand "be yourself." I learned to be as real as I could possibly be, and forgive myself for every mistake I made on the air.

People are going to see the mistakes again and again and again. The challenge has been to forgive myself for not being a perfect yoga teacher. Yoga teachers are not perfect beings, although students like to think of us as such. It's just not true. As a teacher, it was so hard to watch my mistakes, and so-called mistakes on the air are blown up bigger than life. If you are sensitive, you think about people seeing this mistake time and time again.

It forced me to look at the situation we are all in. Patricia Sun, who has been a positive influence on me, said that a mistake is a great opportunity. She is a wonderful spiritual teacher. It's a "miss take" that you can do again and again until you get it right. Television has been a very great taskmaster. It's been a humongous guru for me.

You discovered yoga through Life *magazine when you were eleven years old in 1947. Did that have an impact on your life?*

When I was thirteen years old, I saw a picture of Ramana Maharshi in *Life* magazine. That moment had a great impact on my life. I had an experience with his energy that totally turned my life around. It is very difficult to explain in words, and I have spent the rest of my life trying to understand it myself.

It's strange how pictures can hold the presence of spiritual beings. There is something captured in their face. It's something I don't understand.

My father died while I was at an *ashram* in Harriman, New York. I was upset, naturally, and I had a long drive home. A friend brought out a picture of Ramana Maharshi. I had not read many of his works, because they were so over my head I couldn't possibly understand them. My friend said, "Sit with the picture for a moment, get calmed down and centered, and then go home." I did what is called *trataka*, or gazing at the picture. Ramana Maharshi had such a wonderful face and compassionate eyes it was no problem at all. I sat with this picture and a voice said, "Close your eyes."

From that meditation experience, I can tell you I really do *know* I am not this body, nor am I the mind. None of us has to be afraid of death. We absolutely exist beyond this body. That awareness has been with me the rest of my life. The exciting part is that I know you and I are not alone on this planet. There is always help from other dimensions. You are a child of the Divine. Be up and doing, because life is very short. It's a small amount of time. This is not your eternity.

I was watching the evening news quite a few years ago and wondering about reincarnation. Everything in the evening news was carnage. I was thinking, "Reincarnation? Who would want to come back to this veil of tears? Who in their right mind would want to come back?" Then a very strong voice said, "You chose to come back." It was like a bolt of lightning. It shook me to my bones. I said to myself, "But I feel so fearful here, and I am very unhappy." This voice said with great compassion, "You have all the tools you need."

Why did you start practicing yoga?

My doctor recommended I try yoga. I was a fairly athletic young woman until I had two children. I wasn't sleeping well. My back was in pain. I was kind of smoking.

Kind of *smoking!*

Kind of smoking. But the worst part was the mantle of sadness I constantly carried. I could hardly articulate that part, because I didn't know it myself. I was deeply sad. Yoga helped me out of my sadness, my depression.

Yoga postures massage muscles and emotions held within them. What the mind has forgotten, the body remembers long after. Our old memories and old "stuckness" is hidden in our musculature. As you begin to do the postures, a lot of that quietly dissolves and is released. Often people will feel deep memories and tears from stuff that has been hidden behind the shoulder blades or within the chest. It just releases on its own.

Did the practice resonate with you?

It resonated from the moment I realized I was going to have to practice. I hated the stiffness I felt the day after a yoga class or going to class unprepared. I made the choice to practice. As soon as you begin to study yoga, something changes. It might be your choice not to continue. As soon as I began to practice, my body began to change and so did my outlook on life. I began to feel better.

Yoga led me to classes in New York City with *swamis* who were coming from India. That led me to *ashrams*. *Ashrams* led me to meeting Swami Chidananda, President of the Divine Light Society at the Sivinanda Ashram in Rishikesh, India. He continues to inspire me.

How has Swami Chidananda influenced you?

One day, my husband, Bob, and I were boating on Long Island Sound, and we were caught in a dense fog. He's a great navigator. I was sitting at the front of the boat listening for bells and buoys. I was very relaxed with water all around me. In the blink of an eye something happened in the center of my chest like a thumb push-ing against me. There was this huge feeling of intense joy, but also a sweet sadness. It was a longing to go home. This home was spelt *Om*! All I wanted to do was love God and go some place where I could do that. My family was too distracting.

I went to see Swami Chidananda in Val Morin, Canada. I weepingly told him my experience. He was very quiet. Then he said, "It felt like a big thumb pushing from the inside out?" I said, "Yes." I told him I wanted to leave everything and be in adoration of the love of God. He said, "Lilias, you have been called." That was reassuring, because I didn't know what in the world had happened. He went on to say, "But you have been called *after* you were married, not before." I remember feeling disappointed, but actually he was right on. He said, "Go back and get into your family. Take everything you desire—your adoration of God—go back and put it into your children and your family. Put it into your life."

Do you count that among the best advice you have received in life?

I would say that was *the* best advice. I would have gone in the opposite direction.

I like having people reflect on turning points because it is inspiring for everybody. When a student asked me to give my first talk at the Stamford, Connecticut library, I leapt at the chance. I deliberated about what I was going to wear, what postures I was going to do, if I should stand on my head. She never told me who the audience was going to be. I walked into the library on a Sunday evening. I could hear my class chattering away. When I came around the corner, everyone was seated in a wheelchair. That moment was another turning point. The universe was holding a big mirror in front of me saying, "What are you going to do, prance around in your pink leotard or get down to work?"

When did you develop a meditation practice?

Meditation was something I really did not want to do. I absolutely did not like it, but I was going to *ashrams* and they required you to sit your buns down for half-an-hour or longer. It was truly the last thing on my list, but at a certain point, my dreams directing me to meditate got so loud I had to listen. I started, dragging my feet, a minute at a time, two minutes at a time. There was not a more antsy individual to sit next to during meditation than me. I had tremendous agitation, but for some reason, I stuck with it.

I was taught very good relaxation techniques. I had very good teachers. *Yoga-nidra* was part of my study. It is a deep process—rather painful actually. It is painful lying on the floor for an hour in *savasana*. Someone guides you through relaxation, starting with your little toe. The mind freaks out. Everything erupts. It can be very uncomfortable, but I am very grateful for that kind of training, because the results go inward. I also understand when it happens to my students.

Do you meditate daily?

Oh yeah, twenty minutes to a half-an-hour. It's a daily requirement.

Why?

The mind gets awfully cluttered, crowded, and talky. After meditation, all the chattiness quiets down. Also, you are growing in consciousness, confidence, and maturity. You are much more open to whatever comes. The inner eye opens. The inner ears open. You become much more attentive to whom you are meeting and their energy, what you are saying, and what you can do for someone in the moment.

Describe your personal practice.

I do personal practice in the morning. It can be as short as twenty minutes, or it can be as long as two hours. My practice consists of spiritual reading, contemplation, meditation, and physical practice. That's just very important.

I consider two days a week of weight training to be very much a part of my practice. Your physical and spiritual muscles need stretching and strengthening every day. I feel like I am missing something if I don't do it.

Are you involved in church?

I enjoy going to all churches. I appreciate the words of Christ, and I am inspired by Christ. I enjoy communion. I love the idea of what it symbolizes, and I put my whole self into it. I was born a Christian, not a Buddhist. Although I appreciate Buddhism tremendously, Christianity is in my bones.

Do you ever ponder your legacy?

I was sitting with my grandson as he was reading and thinking, "What sort of a world am I leaving these precious children? By the time they reach college, I will be in the latter part of my life. Maybe I will see them married. Life is moving on so quickly. What sort of a world am I going to leave them? A world that is so fraught with uncertainty, pain, and questions."

The impression that quietly came to my own awareness was that you do the inner work of clearing away spaces, so your soul can expand and bloom. You come to know yourself as the light you truly are. That takes spiritual elbow grease. It takes inner work. That kind of elbow grease will be felt in your family. It will live on after you for generations to come and make a huge difference in your family unit today. It will make a huge difference in a larger sense, in the evolution of the human race. The work we do, the conversations with people on airplanes—looking into people eyes, saying thank you, being generous, polite, caring, and loving without asking anything in return—truly make a difference. It is going to make a difference in the next hundred years. This inner scrubbing is very important.

How does one practice inner scrubbing?

I think a wonderful place to start is with the seed-word grateful. I have noticed how grateful has come into our mainstream vocabulary far more since Oprah Winfrey mentioned keeping a journal of what you are grateful for. Grateful is a wonderful ancient word to think about. It has a sweet, warm energy to it that is very close to love.

Also, practicing hatha yoga is wonderful. Hatha yoga shears away and melts away and dissolves the stress and strain we don't even know we are carrying. All of a sudden the spirit, the energy, the sweetness, rises to the top with ease. Then one can move into relaxation and breath, then into meditation. There are as many directions on how to meditate as there are people who ask the question. Once the mind is focused, you learn how to quiet the monkey mind and tune in to a still place. Learning how to experience relaxation is so important.

The heart connection has been something I have had no trouble cultivating a taste for. Adoration comes easily to me. As you walk along the path of yoga, life opens you up to wisdom and a discerning balance of heart and mind. There is an energy that comes with that. It's a powerful sweetness and nothing satisfies it except that experience. The taste begins to cultivate and you can return, again and again, in meditation, in relaxation, and in yoga postures. In my own practice, I begin the day that way and end the day that way. If I don't have a heart/mind connection, I feel remorse and sadness, and I am deeply bereft.

The heart connection is always there. I leave it to have a tiff with my husband or get mad on the highway. But then I realize that something is missing. The heart center that we speak about is in the right side of our chest. The physical heart to the left side, but there is truly a heart center in every human being. The heart *chakra* as it's called is not dissectable, so it is hard for the medical community to understand. As we are developing as humans, we are developing a spiritual heart. When this truly happens, how can we possibly kill anything or anyone?

Does this heart connection give you the sense of a higher being involved in our lives?

Yes, there is no place where God is not. One of my teachers, Jean Houston, says, "You recognize the God in hiding in another being." As we expand and deepen our consciousness, we are able to see and accept it with more confidence. You recognize there is a light in the other being. I am becoming, day by day, much quicker in recognizing this. I feel it with more comfort.

We are really divine beings of light, or *atman*. Daily we experience what it's like to be a human being and spiritualize every aspect of that being. If I look at my life that way, then I can forgive. It makes life far more expansive. I don't have to be doing anything glamorous, because life is a fascinating journey and the only moment is now.

Lilias Folan has been described by *Yoga Journal* as "one of the most influential people in yoga in the twentieth century." For fifteen years, she was the host of *Lilias, Yoga and You*, which was nationally syndicated to 260 PBS stations from 1970 – 1985. She later created a 52-part hatha yoga series entitled *Lilias!*, which ran on PBS from 1987 – 1996. She has appeared on *Good Morning America*, *Today*, and *Donahue*, and has been interviewed by *Time*, *People*, and *TV Guide*. Her first book, *Lilias, Yoga and You* has sold over 500,000 copies.

Lilias attended Bennington College where she studied painting, drawing, and the Italian language in Rome. She began her yoga practice in 1964 and studied with Swami Vishnu-devananda of the Sivananda lineage. In 1973, she traveled to India to study Vedanta philosophy and meditation under the tutelage of Swami Chidananda of the Divine Light Society in Rishikesh. She continued meditation practice with Swami Muktananda and has studied hatha yoga with T.K.V. Desikachar and B.K.S. Iyengar.

Lilias serves on the board of numerous yoga associations and continues to teach internationally. The mother of two sons and grandmother lives in Cincinnati with her husband, Bob.

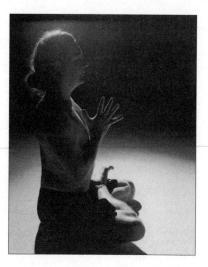

ERICH SCHIFFMANN

LOS ANGELES

You are one of the few yoga teachers I have met who began practicing yoga as a teenager.

Most people who start young don't keep doing it. I know people who started at that age. They found the poses very easy and were not challenged enough. After a few years, they stopped. I'm one of the few people who started early and kept doing it. Part of what's kept me in the game is teaching. Teaching has been a large part of what yoga has been about for me. It's definitely been part of my *sadhana*. A big part of my learning is getting in front of a group and trying to be clear. I know if I weren't teaching there would have been periods when I didn't do any yoga. Maybe I would have stopped all together. Teaching has kept me in there.

When you teach, your practice changes radically because you're no longer doing it for yourself only. Demonstrating communicates a meaning. Touching somebody communicates a meaning. But a large part of teaching is being able to put into words this essentially non-verbal activity. It's made me more self-observant in my personal practice. Teaching is not just telling people what to do, but watching closely and seeing if they're taking in what's being suggested. Trying to sense whether they're being receptive to it or resisting it. And then changing my M.O. in the moment in order to increase their willingness to stay with it as much as possible. I'm learning by teaching.

How do you encourage a student who may be resisting?

People start resisting when they are making themselves do something that they don't really want to be doing. They are there because they think they should be there, or they're comparing themselves to somebody next to them. They're pushing themselves too hard. Actually, it's a healthy response to be resisting, if you're pushing yourself too hard. I try to diminish any sort of comparison happening in the class, and encourage people to keep it on the easy side, rather than "no pain, no gain." If I say, "Keep it on the easy side," people will stay on the easy side and then voluntarily nudge into their edges. But if I say, "Really push into your edges," they tend to stay back and not do anything.

What attracted you to yoga?

The surfers I idolized started getting into Meher Baba and Paramahansa Yogananda. I started copying them and doing yoga on the beach before going surfing to be more flexible. I didn't want to do the poses when I first started. I was more interested in the spiritual stuff. The thought of bending over and having to touch my toes wasn't that appealing. In fact, when I saw Iyengar's *Light on Yoga* for the first time I thought, "That's not yoga. It's awfully physical."

Physically, you're a big yogi.

Before I was tall and skinny, now I'm tall and filled out.

It's impressive to see flexibility at your size.

I hear that a lot. You usually don't see a big guy capable of doing certain poses. *Asana* is easier if you're thin.

Were you athletic growing up?

I was very athletic. I was into baseball and surfing—especially surfing. Being out on the water first thing in the morning and last thing at night, watching the sunset, was a very spiritual thing. Surfers are spiritual in a surprising way. When the surfers are waiting for waves, no one's talking. I didn't even realize this until years later. There will be ten or twenty guys just sitting. It's unusual for a group of people to be involved with something and not talking. It's meditative.

Did you become totally immersed in yoga once the bug bit?

Yeah, bam! I'm still totally bit.

Has it been your only profession?

When I was a teenager I delivered pizza and sold beauty supplies. Those are the only other jobs I've had. I went to Krishnamurti's high school, Brockwood Park, in England and took my first yoga lessons with a student of Desikachar's. I was twenty-one when I started teaching.

You must have found Krishnamurti's Think on These Things *very compelling.*

Absolutely.

It made you go to an extra year of high school. Not many kids say, "Give me the fifth year!"

I didn't have to take the exams.

How did you discover this life-changing book?

My best friend, Bob Ackerman, read it, gave it to me and said, "This is the best book I've ever read. You've got to check it out." Because Bob was giving it to me, I looked at it seriously. It was very philosophical, but rounded, intelligent, and poetic. It helped me to start making sense out of life. It made life seem mystical, wondrous, with a purpose. I started reading all his books. They were the only things I read for a number of years. When I heard he started a high school in England, I thought, "I've got to go there," even though I had just finished high school.

In high school, I would hitchhike to Ojai where Krishnamurti gave public talks. I would take a sleeping bag, climb over somebody's fence, and sleep in their backyard in order to hear Krishnamurti. It was fun. I was so taken by his teachings. He was a handsome guy, courteous, spoke well, and was interested in profound things. He was in his mid-seventies by the time I met him, but still very vital and at the height of his powers. He was totally appealing.

Someone had given Krishnamurti a big mansion in the countryside of southern England to be his retirement home. He said, "I don't need a mansion. I'll take this wing, and why don't we make a school out of the rest of it?" When I went, there were twenty-five students and thirty staff members. He was there for a couple of months out of the year. The rest of the year he traveled. Whenever possible, I sat next to him at lunch and talked to him.

The school was set up so Krishnamurti wouldn't be the main focal point, and the school wouldn't become dependent on him. His whole teaching was "Become your own light, don't depend on me, don't depend on any authority. Go into yourself, figure it out, and be a light unto yourself."

Was there a sense of awe?

Yeah. He was incredible. But he was approachable and friendly, and tried not to encourage the sense of awe.

What led you to India?

Krishnamurti had suggested I go there. That's why I went. India was interesting. I was twenty when I went. I was excited, but scared. I didn't know anybody there. I remember the sounds, the smells, the people, the heat, the incense, the flowers, the beauty, and the ugliness, all in the first glance. It was such strong sensory stimulation. My first thought was "I came *here* to learn yoga?" It felt filthy. It was a beautiful, filthy place. It seemed like an odd place to come halfway around the world to. It made me realize that people there are totally oblivious to what's going on here, and people here are oblivious to what's going on there. Everyone is in their own little world.

You studied with Desikachar. Describe that experience.

He was a fairly new teacher, but he had been teaching Krishnamurti. I would go into his room, and we would sit down. He started
asking me if I liked living in India, did I like the food, how was it living near the beach, do you like the humidity, things like that. He
would tell me about his life, and I would look at my watch. A half an
hour had gone by and I would think, "I've only got half an hour left.
When are we going to start the yoga." Then I realized that he wasn't
going to spoon-feed me. When I asked him a question about yoga, he
started becoming generous with the information. It was unusual,
because in school I was used to being crammed full of information.
There it was, "If you want to know something, ask a question."

At first I thought it was strange. But then I started liking it,
because it made me come up with my questions. What did I want to
know? Why was I here? At that time, I had no thought of becoming
a yoga teacher. I just wanted to learn yoga.

Krishnamacharya, Desikachar's father, was always sitting on the
porch in a little wicker chair. I would ride up on my bike, walk up,
and give him the *namaste*. No response. *Ever*. He would see me do
it. And other people would do it. No response. I'm not really sure
what that was about. He was in his eighties when I knew him, met
him, *saw* him. I didn't know the guy!

When you were unacknowledged by him.

Yeah, unacknowledged by him. Physically, he was beautiful.
He was perfect, except his two front teeth were missing. I heard
Krishnamacharya say three things. [*speaking in a monotone voice*]
"Your teacher is not here today." "Please lock your bi-cycle."
"Yoga is not mechanical."

Yoga is not mechanical.

That was great. He didn't say that to me. I overheard him say that to somebody.

You lost a friend in India.

My friend died. He got hepatitis, turned yellow, and smelled bad. He tried to cure himself naturalpathically. It seemed like it had worked. All the symptoms went away. We thought, "It works!" A few weeks later it came back with a vengeance. It was a horrible death. The liver filters out poisons. When it's not doing that, your brain gets poisoned. His speech became slurred. He had a hard time walking. I got sick. I was in the hospital. He was in the hospital. He died. I thought, "That's me in two weeks." I was so sick I didn't even care. I was tired and lethargic. It wasn't painful. Death wasn't scary. It was more like, "So?" I wrote a letter to my mother saying, "No pain. You were great. See you later."

Did that shape you?

I have definite views about death now, which I didn't have then.

Would you care to share them?

My view at the moment is that death isn't real. There isn't such a thing. Death seems so real, because you see everybody dying. When you meditate and do yoga and feel the energy that we are made of, the experience is that life is an ongoing renewal. That changed the way I do my life. Up until I was thirty, in the back of my mind there was always this thought: "Why bother doing such and such a thing? You're just going to die anyway. Why bother learning spiritual things? You're just going to die anyway." There didn't seem to be any point, because I was just going to die anyway.

Then it hit me—you don't "just die anyway." Life is ongoing. *Now* became more meaningful and important. Meditation started taking on more significance. Rather than just being a stress reduction technique, it became more meaningful, mysterious, and interesting.

You don't consider yourself an Iyengar teacher.

They don't either!

So, it's mutual! Iyengar teachers express a deep devotion to Mr. Iyengar.

I understand their devotion, because he's a brilliant man. When someone is communicating something as well as he is, you're grateful. If you watch him practice, it's not mechanical. He's being creative. He's not telling himself what to do, the way those of us who learn from him start doing. He's sensing inwardly, and then talking about it to others, trying to give them clues on how to find a good energy flow. He's very creative in his practice. I think he's a beautiful man.

When you're a beginner, it's really helpful to have concrete clues. Rotate your arm this way, stretch this skin that way, so that you begin to get an inner sense of what to do. The problem comes when you've memorized all the rules and you start thinking that's the only way to do it. The real practice is to find the new feeling of rightness, which might involve rotating your arm slightly differently or stretching the skin in the opposite direction.

When he would say, "Move your skin this way," and I would, there was an inner *ding!* The thing to do on your own is to look for the inner *ding* or feeling of rightness. Then you're doing your yoga, because you're following the inner sense of what feels right, rather than doing something that was imposed externally. At first, it's helpful to do that. I did it like that for years. But then I started resisting, because it started feeling like a chore rather than a joy. When I got the inner sense of how to do it, I understood where he was coming up with all this information. It was going with the flow.

I talk about moving into stillness, so that you can be quiet enough and open enough to be guided from within. That's what the inner teacher is. It's the wave listening to the ocean. The function of the teacher is to help someone do that, rather than become devoted to the teacher.

Describe your perception of stillness.

When people hear the word stillness, they think of motionless. Stillness is like a perfectly centered top that is spinning so fast it appears motionless. If the top is not perfectly centered, it will appear erratic. If it is not spinning fast enough, you will detect the movement. Stillness is this perfectly centered top that has so much energy and so much harmony that it's not in conflict with itself. The feeling tone of it is harmonious, joyful, smooth, pleasant. Stillness is getting your mind quiet. When your mind is quiet, you have the clearest perspective on whatever's going on. It's to our advantage to have the clearest perspective available in order to be the most effective. The clearer the view of reality, the less you will suffer and the happier you will be.

Meditation is the main practice in yoga and always has been as far as I can understand. The poses arose out of the centered meditative state. People were meditating and felt moved to move. The poses help you get back into the meditative state and sustain the meditative state. In class, I begin with meditation, do the poses, then relaxation as long as possible, and end with meditation. If you can get people to be quiet in the now, spontaneous education starts to occur. When you have the quiet mind, intuitive revelation flows in. The intuitive revelation you get is spiritual teachings that are pertinent to you, much more pertinent than reading a great spiritual book. It's like opening a window, so the breeze can come through. I don't have to make the breeze.

You're letting the flow flow. You start trusting that more. You start trusting your deepest feelings, whether you can explain them or not. Before I wouldn't let myself do something unless I could explain it. Now the explanation can come later.

Dare to do as you are prompted to do. From experience, we know that when you trust the deeper sense, it flows in miraculous ways. Things are put together in such an amazing order that you couldn't have done by yourself.

Does this give you the sense of a loving energy?

Absolutely. Every specific thing is a wave on the ocean of consciousness. Every wave is a specific expression of the Infinite. When you as a wave meditate and sink into yourself, you start feeling the depths of the ocean as being the truest thing about who you are. That alone changes your self-concept, because you're no longer just a specific little wave bobbing around on the surface. If there's a wave, there's got to be an ocean, being the source of who you are.

The Sanskrit word is *satchidananda*. *Sat* means Being or existence, *chit* means Consciousness or Mind, and *ananda* means bliss. Three separate words. You roll them together and the idea is that the feeling tone of Being is Consciousness, which is blissful. You can prove it by relaxing into yourself and staying with your actual now experience. You start feeling the joy of being. You are surrounded by this thing and loved by this thing. And you are this thing in specific expression. That's radical.

When you sink into yourself, start experiencing your true mind and nature, and look out and see other waves, you start seeing the very same ocean in them that you've become familiar with within yourself. Whereas before, you would look out and see others, potentially hostile, and contract in order to protect yourself. Now your personal experience would be that the world is a less fearful place to be, because you're not seeing alien energies the way you used to. You are seeing aspects of yourself, which is good. In *your* seeing it in them, you help bring it out of them.

Krishnamurti was a big influence in that way, and my mother was a big influence in that way. If you're behaving like a single, isolated, egotistical wave, they see through that and love you anyway. The reason why people like Krishnamurti are so great, is because they can see through the persona that you're presenting as yourself, to the ocean that's got to be there if there's a specific wave, and start relating to that thing which is really the most real about you. Relating to that helps bring it out and confirms it in your own mind. There's only this one infinite thing going on. There's only one Self, one Infinite Presence. That's what we are.

When you become still enough to sink into the ocean, what you feel is the pulse of the ocean, or ongoing creation. It's not dead, motionless, lacking inspiration. It's the opposite. You feel inspired to do things from a creative place.

You were interested in art and being an artist. Is that a part of who you are now?

No, but a similar impulse comes up. I have a strong desire to write in the same way that teaching is part of my *sadhana*. I never really use that word in my own mind, but it works. My house has a flat roof, and I'll go up and meditate on the roof with my Sony tape recorder. I just sit and meditate. After a while, ideas flow through and I speak them into the tape recorder. A lot of my book was written that way. I catch it on tape.

It started happening years ago when I was falling asleep. I would get this quick insight about something. It would usually come in a quick sentence. It would be this great idea or answer to something. I would think, "I'll write that down in the morning." And in the morning, I would have no idea what it was. I would get frustrated, because I knew I had lost something that I thought had some meaning. I got to the point where I would get up and speak one or two sentences into a tape recorder. Then suddenly there would be more sentences and I would end up with a paragraph. I didn't feel like I was making it up. I felt like I was being taught by something beyond me, and yet it was coming from within me.

When do you do your roof meditation?

It's usually between eleven at night and three in the morning. The next day I transcribe it. If there are holes, somehow when transcribing, I get back in that same sphere and I flesh it out, complete the idea, or add to it. Sometimes I write it by hand, sometimes I type it, and sometimes I speak it. Whichever feels like it's going to work the best at that time. When that first started happening, if I didn't use a pen to write it down, I couldn't hear it as well. But the moment I started writing it down, it completed the circuit. I can look back and see by the handwriting what state I was in. It's a place of humility, because it's not you doing it. You're being the student.

When do you practice yoga?

On an ideal day, I do yoga from ten till noon, then again in the evening. Lately, however, I've been doing it mostly in the evenings from six to eight.

Are you not a morning person?

I am not a morning person. I used to get up and make myself practice at six in the morning. But I'm more an evening person. Left to my own devices I go to bed a little later every night. For a number of years, I was in a situation where I could do that. It was fun to not have to be regimented with a schedule.

Many people say you must practice in the morning.

I think you should be sensitive to the time when you feel like you really want to be doing it, when you're hungry for it. There usually is a moment in the day when you feel like doing yoga or you feel like doing meditation. Rather than being too scheduled about it, be sensitive to those moments.

One of the reasons people cite for morning practice is that if you do it at the beginning of the day there's nothing to interfere. If you wait until later in the day, your practice may evaporate because of other obligations, or you may procrastinate and simply not do it.

If that's happening, it's a good idea to discipline yourself to fit it in. Otherwise, the discipline is to be sensitive to when the moment is right. Then you're not making yourself do something just because everyone else is saying you've got to do it first thing in the morning. I was hassling myself with that for years. In the beginning, if I took a day off, I didn't know if I would keep doing yoga. Now I know that I'll keep doing it. So if I need to take a day off, I can do it without guilt tripping myself. It's actually a yogic thing to do—to be sensitive to the fact that today's not the day. That's more yogic than making yourself do it when you don't want to, when it's not the right thing to be done.

Any closing thoughts?

I'm not familiar with the *sutras* and all the various texts, though I've read bits and pieces. I'm not well versed in the literature of yoga. Partly from Krishnamurti's influence. I'm glad, because the whole emphasis is dive into yourself and find out what your experience is. When I come up with something and I then see it in the *Vedas*, it's confirmation rather than me adopting that stance. I don't want to brainwash myself into a belief system in advance, because I don't know if it's right. I don't want to dupe myself. I *do* want to find out what's really going on. I *do* want to experience what's true. You can sink into your quiet mind and be taught from within. Dive into yourself and let the ocean teach you. That's the main thing. The universe is on your side, because you are the universe in specific expression.

Erich Schiffmann began practicing yoga as a teenager over thirty years ago. At age eighteen, he was a student at J. Krishnamurti's high school, Brookwood Park, in England. After a year-and-a-half in India, studying with T.K.V. Desikachar and B.K.S. Iyengar, he returned to Brookwood Park, where he taught yoga for five years. His most influential mentor is respected yoga instructor Joel Kramer. His award-winning, best-selling video, *Yoga Mind and Body*, featuring Ali McGraw, has sold more than 250,000 copies. Erich is a contributing writer for *Yoga Journal* and the author of *Yoga: The Spirit and Practice of Moving into Stillness*. He teaches yoga in Los Angeles and travels internationally, conducting workshops, retreats, and teacher trainings.

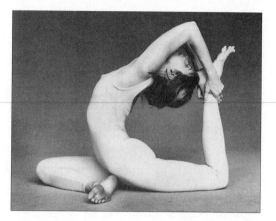

PATRICIA WALDEN

BOSTON

You were my first yoga teacher. I started practicing with your Yoga Journal's Practice for Beginners video. I put it in my VCR and was immediately intimidated and inspired by your demonstration in Death Valley.

It's an extraordinary place. You should go there. It was five in the morning, and a camera crew of about twenty trekked into the desert in the dark. When the sun came up there were purple clouds around, because there was going to be a big storm. That special light lasted for about ten minutes. Fortunately, my body was warmed up, and I captured what I wanted. It was a perfect five minutes. It was wonderful.

The landscape inspired me to move. Yesterday, when I was doing backbends during a photo shoot, looking out at the sky and seeing the wide-open space helped me to open my lungs and chest. I can absorb space I see on the outside and internalize it. But the desert was more than that. Not only this vast sky, but the beauty was so inspiring that I was having a beyond-body experience. I was energy. It was extraordinary.

How were you selected for the video?

I had to fly to Santa Monica and teach a spontaneous class in a city park. It was really fascinating. First of all, when you are performing and teaching, you are not terribly relaxed, especially when there's traffic going by and kids playing. As I was teaching, Steve Adams, the owner of Living Arts and producer of the video, wasn't looking at me. He was looking away from me with his hands in his pockets. I thought, "Well, I guess this isn't going very well. I don't think he particularly cares for me." He acted disinterested throughout the whole thing. Afterwards, he came up to me and said, "That was absolutely fabulous. That was extraordinary. This is just what I'm looking for." I was completely shocked because the message his body was giving me was totally different.

What role does age play in a yoga practice?

People in their twenties and early thirties have minds that are different than someone who is in their late thirties, forties, or fifties. At a certain point in your life, you have more desire to penetrate inward, to reflect inward, and to achieve stillness. Younger people really love yoga, but they like the movement. They want to do something that has a spiritual connection, something that's heartfelt, but they need to move. For most people, the quietness and the stillness comes later in life. I have been watching over the last five or six years. I look at people who do Iyengar yoga in a serious way and most of them are in their late thirties, forties, fifties, or sixties. Younger people don't want a teacher who says, "Come watch." They don't want to come watch. They want to do.

B.K.S. Iyengar's philosophy is that you must penetrate your being. He really wants us to understand how different actions in one pose fit together. You must be mindful. You are not just coming into the pose, inhaling, exhaling, holding for four breaths, and coming up. He wants you to feel how your arm relates to your shoulder. When you extend your arms to the maximum, he wants you to ask how it feels in your lungs. What is the feeling in your eyes? What is the feeling in your brain? What is the feeling in your feet? It's an external and internal journey. You are reflecting on what's going on outside and what's going on inside.

Iyengar wants consciousness to grace your entire being. It's not just holding a pose and waiting until it's over. Instead, it's really penetrating from your outer sheath, which is the physical body, to your psychological body. All the eight limbs of yoga are in one pose, if you do the pose with the particular attitude—mindfulness. It's really a meditation. You're doing it wholeheartedly, one-pointed. Iyengar calls it *ekagrata* state. Can I exist in my big toe? Can I exist in my lungs? Can I exist in my eyes? Can I exist in my ears? You really explore each part of the body in the pose.

The first workshop I ever attended was with Rodney Yee. He said, "Press down your baby toe." I tried, but nothing moved.

There wasn't intelligence there. Iyengar would say your toe has a mind. You hadn't awakened the mind, or the intelligence, of your baby toe.

The philosophy behind this is that you can't know your inner Self, the *atman*, if you don't know your outer sheath, the body. We learn to find ourselves by first finding and then knowing our own body, by understanding how my toes work, how my hands work. Why do the toes spread so freely on my right foot, but not on my left? It's easier to understand something you can see, rather than something you can't see. You learn in a gross way first. Then the journey goes inward from the gross to the subtle.

Do you have to conquer your physical body to fully delve into your spiritual body?

I wouldn't call it conquer. I would say understand it. I love physical challenges. Some people love doing *asana,* but they don't like challenges. I love the challenge of doing a new pose. I decided years ago I wanted to do every pose in *Light on Yoga.* To find yourself, you don't have to do every pose in *Light on Yoga.* That's not necessarily going to bring you closer to yourself. My own experience has been that doing poses I never thought were possible, working through the tightness in my body and building strength, has brought me confidence, self-esteem, and power. It's more than conquering the body. Going to the unknown and doing things I never thought I was capable of doing have made me tremendously confident.

If you had a lot of fear as a child, you weren't athletic, and you didn't hang upside down on jungle gyms or do cartwheels, and then as an adult you are able to go upside down and do a full-arm balance for three minutes, you can change your consciousness. That is incredibly powerful. It's liberating. You would think that would stop at the physical plane, but it seeps into many layers of your being. You start to feel differently about yourself, and then people start responding to you differently.

I see so clearly in my students how the practice of *asana* builds self-esteem and makes them feel adequate. People in America suffer from low self-esteem and most people I meet feel inadequate. Maybe it's universal, but I see it so much in the United States.

Doing *asana* and doing *savasana* builds self-esteem. It makes you feel adequate, because it's an incredible form of self-care. When you learn to care for yourself, it really changes the way you relate to people. It's a wonderful gift that a yoga teacher can give a student— to help them realize they are adequate and full.

You are incredibly flexible. What was your level of flexibility when you started yoga?

I wouldn't say I was flexible. I was loose. Flexible is healthy. I didn't have control. There wasn't a balance of flexibility and strength. Strength came slowly. I can now stand on my hands for five minutes. It took me a year to learn handstand, because my arms were not strong. Building strength in my body has been toughest for me. When I first started doing yoga, I could do *uttanasana* and *upavistha konasana*. But I didn't have strength in my arms to do a full-arm balance or push up into a backbend.

How did you get into yoga?

I started reading books about yoga when I was ten. I was unusual in that at a very early age I had yearnings for God. I was always looking for manifestations of God. I remember writing notes to God as a child when I had questions that Mommy and Daddy couldn't answer, and imagining that He was answering me in different ways, like through the sun coming out. When I became a teenager, those yearnings departed for a while. In my late teens, they came back again. I was a sixties child. I feel very fortunate that I was a teenager and a young adult during the sixties, because that time was so good for questioning life.

I grew up in Newton, Massachusetts, but I went to college at San Francisco State and got distracted by the sixties stuff. I was feeling lost and empty. I had these yearnings, and I had a certain awakening, but I didn't have a medium for it. I was involved for some time with a Sufi master called Sam Lewis. He taught Sufi dancing and Sufi meditation. He was my first spiritual teacher, and he had an extraordinary influence on my life. He called his dances "dances for universal peace." He introduced me to meditation. A seed was planted. He died about three years after I met him. I had feelings of emptiness and longing again. I tried many different things. I won't give you the long list, but since it was the sixties you can imagine. They gave me temporary fullness.

I was dancing a lot, and I always felt good when I was dancing. One day, the teacher brought in a yoga teacher to show us some relaxation techniques. At that time, I was reading existentialist authors. They made the empty feelings even worse, and I got away from them quickly. So I was already in this place where I was searching. I remember my first yoga pose I ever did—the shoulderstand. I thought, "This feels so familiar. I've done this before." I felt like I was coming home to something. For the first time I felt this wonderful feeling of fullness. It was extraordinary. That was a turning point in my life, although I didn't become a serious practitioner at that time. I found something I had been looking for a long, long time in the shoulderstand.

My interest in yoga had nothing to do with physical stuff. In the sixties, we weren't really embodied. We were more in our minds and wanting to change our consciousness. Physical fitness was not happening then. My interest was in seeking enlightenment and finding a way to feel peaceful inside. That was my attraction to *asana*.

Did you begin taking classes?

Sporadically. I was young—twenty-one. I was still searching, and I tried different kinds of yoga. I really loved the yoga, but I wasn't consciously looking for a teacher. When I look back, I realize had I found a teacher, I would have started practicing earlier. Some people don't need a teacher. I really needed someone to ignite me.

In my late twenties, I finally met Iyengar. That was another turning point in my life. It was a real case of love at first sight. I met this man, and I immediately knew he was going to change my life. His eyes. The unexplainable. Some people have this tremendous light. There is something about the person that inspires you. Not their words, not their actions, but something about their presence is tremendously powerful. That happened to me. I met him in May of 1976. That following January, I went to India and I have been going every year since.

How long do you stay?

One or two months. I feel so lucky, especially as I get older. It was meaningful to have met a master. Not just a teacher, he's a master. As I get older, I feel so much gratitude to have met a master in this lifetime that suits me so well. It's really extraordinary. Some people can go through their lives wanting to find a teacher, but never finding that person. I am so fortunate that I met someone who has really taken me on. I have a really wonderful relationship with him. When I go to Pune, even when he's not teaching (and he doesn't teach much anymore), I practice with him. He was the lighthouse. He brought me to myself.

How did you meet?

He was doing a tour of the United States. It was his second visit. In the seventies, yoga was just becoming popular. It was the time when people who grew up in the sixties and took drugs realized, "If I keep doing these drugs I might not live very long. All my brain cells are going to get fried."

A lot of people like me did LSD for spiritual experience. We were reading Alan Watts and Aldous Huxley and were really interested in the transformation of consciousness. We thought, "Yoga can do this, too." We discovered that it did, although we had to work for it. The difference is yoga requires discipline.

Were you teaching when you met Iyengar?

I am embarrassed to say I was. I say I am embarrassed because I was self-taught. Today teacher training is very common, but when I started doing yoga in Cambridge, Massachusetts there were only a couple of teachers around. There was no place you could go and learn yoga, so I studied books. There were a few people around that had been doing yoga longer than me. I went to their classes. I really loved it. There was nothing I had ever enjoyed as much as doing yoga.

One day I decided, "I think I'll try teaching this." I taught a class in the Adult Center for Education in Boston. There were thirty people in the class, and I was paid nine dollars. I was still living in the sixties mentally, and I shunned money. I thought it was more important to do something meaningful that you loved to do. I didn't care about the money. I would have done it for free. When I think back—nine dollars! Thirty people and nine dollars a class!

When I think of the students that I taught in those days, I think, "Thank God they survived my teaching." I was an inspired teacher, and I loved what I did, but I didn't have a clue about how the body worked. I could demonstrate poses. I could talk about the essence of yoga. I had the feeling, but not a lot of understanding and refinement.

When did teaching become your livelihood?

I started making money at yoga in my early thirties. I have never had a nine-to-five job. I did a little waitressing here and there. I modeled and made a little money dancing. In the sixties, I lived in communal situations, so I didn't need a lot of money to live.

The age of thirty-six was a turning point for me. As I talk to other people, especially women, I see that is a turning point for them, too. I married when I was thirty-five and got divorced when I was thirty-six. That was a big one in my life. I really wanted the marriage to work. The man I was married to didn't like the idea that I had something in my life I really loved. He thought we would get married, and I would stay at home and do the wife thing. That was not me—I had never done anything traditional. The traditional path has not worked for me. I tried and it didn't work. We ended our marriage.

At that time, my relationship to yoga, though I loved it, was mediocre. I wasn't realizing my potential. After my marriage ended, I reached a low point in my life. I had moved out of my home. I remember sitting in my apartment and thinking, "You know, Patricia, you're either going to give this up, or you're going to do it wholeheartedly and give everything you have to this art." I decided that day to devote my life to yoga and that was a real turning point for me. That's when my practice really took off. My practice was okay before, but I had stuff going on in my life that I let interfere. It was during that period that I believe I had an awakening.

At the end of *Light on Yoga*, Iyengar talks about all the arm balances. Those were hard for me. I've always loved taking on something that is difficult. It is a form of *tapas*. You think, "I'm not going to be able to do this," but you make yourself. You say, "I know I'm going to feel so good after I complete this." One day I said to myself, "Go into your yoga room. You're not going to come out until you try every one of those arm balances." That was another turning point.

Iyengar says arm balances require more perseverance than any of the other *asanas*. They are the hardest physically and psychologically. I wasn't able to do them all, but such a wonderful feeling came from taking action. Iyengar says, "Take an action, no matter how small." He's not just talking about doing *asana*. If you feel stuck in your life, if you feel depressed, take an action. Even if it's a tiny action, it can change your consciousness. That was what I did. I knew I wouldn't be able to do those poses, but I could at least try. It's amazing how something like that can change your consciousness, change your feelings about yourself. When I work with people who are depressed, I try to impart that to them.

When you're depressed, the breath doesn't exist in your body. It's shallow. There's no life force moving. I have watched Iyengar work with depressed people. One of the first things he does is say, "Move your eyes up." Just doing that can change your consciousness. I was depressed when I was younger. I thought, "I wish I had met him when I was young." Iyengar gives people who are young and depressed backbends, and he makes them move really fast. "Open your chest. Go and get a block. Move fast. Keep your eyes open. Breathe deeply."

When you walk fast, your life force starts moving. When you do backbends, you're opening your chest. It's really hard to stay depressed if you're doing this action. His whole theory is "take an action, no matter how small." He stays on you, and he's really firm. When you're depressed, often you need somebody who is from the tough-love school of compassion to get you going.

How is your relationship with Iyengar's daughter, Geeta?

In the early days, it wasn't a great relationship. She did not take a liking to me. I think a lot of it was my American image—tall and thin. I really tried to win her love. One time in class, her father was having me demonstrate a pose. Geeta said, "This girl is just a line. You come to India and all the Indian women try to look like you. You're just a line." But over the last five years, she has seen my devotion and my loyalty to *Guruji*. I am there every year. She knows I am sincere and devoted. I am also devoted to her. She is one of my teachers. It was a relationship that I worked for. I had to earn her respect. The same was true with her father, but it took longer with her. Now we have a really wonderful relationship.

Did the Yoga Journal *videos present more opportunities to you?*

The videos presented me with a lot of opportunities that I didn't take advantage of. For example, I had the opportunity to do a television program on public TV in Boston that could have become syndicated. I decided not to do that because it would take me away from my practice. I had a lot of opportunities to be on television and talk shows. I don't like things that take me away from my practice. When I did the videos, I thought, "I'll make enough money so I can take a sabbatical, live in India for a couple of years, and study with Iyengar." I am happiest when I am teaching and practicing by myself at home. I am more of an introvert.

But what about your responsibility to others since you have been placed in a messenger role?

That's a wonderful point. That's what I have been feeling. Although I am trying to do more things like the *Yoga Journal* conference, it goes against my nature. I decided to do more conventions that aren't just Iyengar conventions. I have an opportunity to introduce Iyengar's work to people who might not be introduced to it otherwise. That excites me. Eight years ago, when I first started doing videos, I was leading a very introverted and narrow life. Practice, teaching, practice, teaching. That was an important stage for me to go through—developing my practice and important years of reflection. I feel like I am ready to come out a little more.

What should people be aware of when they practice yoga?

One of the things to remember when you do yoga is that it's very different from other things you do in your life. Eventually, the yoga philosophy should be incorporated into the rest of your life. That will happen on its own. When you are practicing yoga, you want to cultivate an attitude where you are interested in the process, rather than "Can I bring my hands to my feet?," so that it doesn't become like other things you do in your life. What can I learn about myself from this process of trying to bring my hands to my feet? Can I be interested in the emotions that come up in this process? Can I be interested in the sensations in my hamstrings or my quadriceps? The journey of getting there is much more interesting and meaningful than putting your hands to your feet. The journey is the most valuable part.

The brain always wants to dictate. The brain always wants to lead. When you begin a yoga practice, you want to ask your brain to become the distant observer. Let the intelligence of your body rise forth. Let the body's voice lead you into the pose. That's a skill that has to be developed. If you are moving from your brain, there is a very different experience than if you are moving from the voice of your body. Your body has a voice. It's so rich in wisdom, but you have to become quiet to hear that voice. When you reach that place in a pose, you will feel relaxed and refreshed afterwards. Your consciousness will change. If you are working from your brain in a pose, when you finish practicing your body might feel good, but peace of mind isn't there.

What are the benefits of backbends?

They are my favorite poses. Backbends are not beginning poses.

In 1991, Iyengar did a backbend intensive for his senior students. He talked about all the levels of backbending. I'll share some of that with you. First of all, according to him and from my own experience, backbends are the most powerful of all the poses on your nervous system, if they are done correctly. We were talking about depression earlier. There is something about opening your chest and spreading your lungs that has a positive and joyful effect on one's psyche. It's empowering. Backbends done twice a week in an intelligent way, using just the right sequence, can strengthen your nervous system. I can attest to that. When I began yoga, my nervous system was not strong. I was shaky and scattered. My practice of backbends, more than any of the other poses excluding inversions, has strengthened my nervous system.

The way to begin backbends is first to develop strength in your arms and your legs. You get that through dog pose, standing poses, and inversions. Then do supported backbends to open the doors to the armpits. The groin is another set of doors that have to be open.

If you drink a caffeinated beverage, you get a lift. Backbends can give you that lift without the shakiness and without the side effects. It's the physiological effect of the backbend that gets your energy moving, but in a harmonious way. If you do a backbend practice and end with some wonderful full length poses like forward bends, or supine poses like *supta baddha konasana,* when you finish you feel powerful and energized at the same time. Quietness and awareness are running parallel with each other.

Backbends can take the place of drugs for mild depression, if they are done sensibly. I have seen people come out of depression from a good practice of inversions and backbends. Once a week, I do a hundred-and-eight dropovers from *tadasana.* Up and down, up and down, up and down. There is a tremendous feeling of space and joy that comes into your being from that practice. It is really beyond words. It is one of the most extraordinary ways to experience your body as boundless space. That's one of the things back-bends has given me. It doesn't get better than that.

Patricia Walden has been practicing yoga for the past twenty-six years. Her first spiritual teacher was Sam Lewis, a Sufi master that she met in San Francisco in the late 1960s. In 1976, Patricia met B.K.S. Iyengar while he was visiting the United States, and immediately knew she had found her life-long teacher. She travels to Pune, India annually to study with Mr. Iyengar; his son, Prashant; and his daughter, Geeta. She has been teaching yoga for twenty years and has conducted workshops internationally for the past decade. Patricia is the director of the B.K.S. Iyengar Yoga Center of Greater Boston. Her special interests include Sanskrit, yoga for women, and classical Indian music.

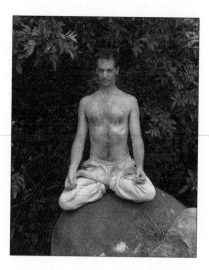

GARY KRAFTSOW

MAUI

What was your introduction to yoga?

My first real experience with yoga was sailing. It's interesting to sail a small boat. You read the wind on the water. You integrate with the winds, the sail, and the rudder. If you integrate everything well, you are a good racer. I see that as the beginning of my yoga.

When I went to high school I did gymnastics and hurt my back. A friend's mother was a yoga teacher. She put me in a posture, rubbed my back, and I got better right away. I wasn't consciously aware that I was getting involved with yoga at this point.

I went into religious studies and that's where I encountered yoga. I discovered Patanjali's *Yoga Sutras*. I really got turned on and spent about six months studying yoga. In 1974, I met a woman who was a yoga teacher and a student of Krishnamacharya. Her husband was chairman of the music department where I went to school. They were taking a study group of dancers and musicians to India. Six months after meeting her I was in India. I went to Krishnamacharya's house and was introduced to him and his son, Desikachar. I became a student of Desikachar.

That's going to the mountaintop pretty quickly.

I was taken there.

Did you experience culture shock when you first traveled to India?

The big shock wasn't when I went to India. It was when I came back to the United States. Suddenly, I saw everything in a totally different light. I realized some of my friends really weren't my friends. I had lost track of popular music. Something shifted for me. You see faith in India. You get a sense of spiritual vitality.

What is your religious heritage?

My ancestors were Jewish. My family entered the United States before the turn of the century. I had a socially Jewish education when I was a kid, but it wasn't a spiritual one.

When I went to undergraduate school I found myself taking classes in religious traditions and philosophy. That was what I was interested in. I saw religion as the cumulative effort of man's attempt at self-understanding. Of course, it's also the cumulative record of man's ignorance and inhumanity. But in the core of the different traditions there is insight into the nature of human experience. What is our purpose here? That was my interest. That's what brought me to yoga. I saw yoga as a methodology of self-investigation and self-discovery that would lead toward self-transformation. The physical aspects were an adjunct.

Did you develop a strong asana practice?

I was a gymnast, so it was easy for me. I could do nearly all the *asanas* when I went to Madras and met Desikachar. I found myself getting more interested in the breath and the spine. Because I had hurt my back, I knew about injury and recovery. My interest with him was more the mind studies, refining and understanding of *asana* practice, how to teach other people, and how to develop *asana* for people with problems. I was more interested in therapeutic application. My own work was about deepening the breath and being able to move the spine in more subtle ways.

Yoga is about the mind. It is not about the body. I was very interested in understanding the nature of the mind and why people suffer. Patanjali, the original codifier of the ancient yoga teachings, is said to have created three traditions—one for the purification of the body, one for the purification of speech, and one for the purification of the mind. The tradition for the purification of the body is *ayurveda*. The tradition for the purification of speech is Sanskrit grammar. The tradition for the purification of the mind is yoga. Implicit in the teachings of yoga is the transformation of the mind. *Asana* is a means to help begin that transformation.

What do you mean by mind?

The mind is the field in which you experience yourself. Mind is the means by which you live. All your perception, all your cognition goes via the mind. The condition of your mind influences how you can function in the world and how you live your life. Yoga is about transforming your mind, so that you can live your life and reach your higher potential, rather than being caught in the dramas of your personality and becoming a victim of external circumstances and acting out the conditioning that you inherited from your parents.

Do we seek clarity of the mind through yoga?

Clarity and discrimination. The ability to see things clearly without distortion from your own motivation. Yoga is overcoming troubling emotional conditions, such as constant frustration or anxiety, and running after things that aren't really important. It is getting in touch with your destiny, your *dharma*.

What is the importance of a teacher?

You need a link with a teacher to help you develop a strong personal practice. Someone who can be a mirror to reflect for you what is important. When I work with students, I don't tell them what's important. I'm just reflecting back to them what's for them.

A teacher helps you maintain a balanced perspective. Growth is not always easy. *Tapas* means many things, but in this context, it's to cook yourself, to purify yourself. It's heat. That takes effort. It's helpful to have a guide, because you can get lost. It's important to have the right guide.

Why does America struggle with the concept of a guru?

There is a confused conditioning in America that comes out of Christianity—that Jesus is the one and only. Any American who rejects the religion of their birth is looking for that one guru who is going to save them. They transfer all this power to the guru. Some gurus are sincere and some gurus are corrupted by the power. Unfortunately, there's a lot of manipulation going on in the guru model.

According to the tradition, a guru is an essential element in transformation, because we're always looking at everything from within where we are. The real meaning of the word guru is "someone who removes darkness." The word *darshan* is important in this context. It comes from the Sanskrit root, *drsya*, which means "to see." Ideally, a guru is reflecting both aspects of yourself—your neurotic self and your transcendent Self—back at you. The idea of the guru is to help the student become the guru.

I was watching PBS when I had an epiphany. An astrophysicist developed the science of getting the Voyager out of the solar system by using the gravitational field of the planets to pick up momentum. Basically, the Voyager would swing around planets like a slingshot. He was explaining the mathematics and the complications. If you don't aim the Voyager toward the planet, it misses. If you aim it too close, it will crash into the planet, or get captured by the gravity and go into orbit.

Many people crash and get absorbed into the mass of the guru. I have seen people get too close to the guru and lose their own identity. Others are sincere devotees of the guru, and they orbit around the guru, rather than using the guru as a means of moving in their own journey and propelling them forward into their own evolution.

That was my first insight. Then I saw the Voyager in relation to psychological problems. Most of us go into orbit around our own self-importance. Our life challenges become the gravity that keeps us locked in orbit around ourselves, but we can use this gravity of personal challenges as a means of growing and moving on in our lives.

Perhaps a guru could have the best of intentions, but the student goes overboard.

That's exactly what Patanjali says. Patanjali warns of the risk of a powerful mind. He says that a powerful mind can influence other minds, but the nature of the influence is dependent on the ego of the individual that is being influenced. Westerners put gurus on a pedestal, find out they are human, and then pull them down.

As a society, we have been cut free from the roots of the past. That brings some benefit. We have a very creative society. But at the same time, most people don't even know what you're talking about when you say "faith." The vast majority of Americans don't have a spiritual foundation, and they are even embarrassed to talk about it.

Many Americans consider yoga a religion.

Yoga is a non-sectarian science of all religion. Yoga is not a religion. Yoga is a methodology. Yoga technology is present in Hinduism, Buddhism, Christianity, and Judaism. Not in the same form, but in the substructures. Patanjali made a systematic presentation of the teachings of religious traditions in a non-sectarian way.

I would like to elevate the understanding of this deep and profound tradition in the West. I would like for people to realize that yoga is not about touching your toes and to appreciate what yoga has to offer in a therapeutic way. We have an obsession with the physical in yoga, which is unfortunate. That is the opposite of yoga.

Can you embrace the spiritual aspects of yoga and still have an hourglass figure?

Absolutely. This body is your temple and you have to take care of it, but the goal isn't to become beautiful. It is important to stay healthy and fit. The ancient science of yoga is also a science of longevity, so you have more time to work out your *karma*. You have more time to work through your confusion and your patterning and become free. Beautiful is not what you look like in the mirror. It's how you are. Beauty is compassion, kindness, joyfulness, and contentment, and cannot be measured by external appearance.

What is yoga therapy?

Yoga therapy is an ancient tradition that begins when a patient recognizes there is a problem and wants to do something about it. If the problem is a physical disease, it may be more about helping the mind come to peace with the condition, or learning how to manage the condition, or actually curing it. It depends upon the disease. Some things we attempt to cure. Some things we don't try to cure. We refer them to other practitioners, but work with the patient in relation to their attitude. In my experience of doing yoga therapy for more than fifteen years, I have had success in conditions ranging from back pain to chronic fatigue to anxiety. Yoga really works.

What is viniyoga?

Viniyoga is a word that has a lot of antecedents. Fifteen years ago, a few of Desikachar's students wanted to know what we should call our yoga. Desikachar asked Krishnamacharya, and he gave the name *viniyoga*. The context is significant, because *viniyoga* teaching comes out of *Nathamuni*—the idea of adapting practices to suit the individual.

A simple way of understanding what we mean by *viniyoga* is that the technology—*asana, pranayama,* chanting, and meditation—should be adapted respecting the needs of the individual to whom they are being applied. It's an ancient understanding, but it's a novel idea in the American yoga world. An *asana* doesn't have one form that everybody should do the same way. The postures are to serve your body. Your body is different than my body. We need to adapt the postures to achieve the desired function in your body.

Viniyoga not only about *asana*. It's about the whole gamut of methodologies or technologies that are applied to effect change in a desired direction. It's not really the name of a lineage as much as a description of our methodology.

What can you share about Desikachar?

He is a brilliant man. Desikachar has a Western education in science, but he studied yoga with his father since he was a baby. His deep interest in yoga comes from watching his father heal people. He graduated at the top of his class in engineering, but he didn't want to be an engineer. He wanted to learn from his father how to help sick people. When Desikachar was in his twenties, J. Krishnamurti came to see Krishnamacharya and he said, "Study with my son." So Desikachar became the yoga teacher of J. Krishnamurti.

J. Krishnamurti was very iconoclastic, and he opposed the whole guru system. He was very much into a radical waking up. J. Krishnamurti invited Desikachar to Switzerland, and that's where he started teaching Westerners. Desikachar is a real master. He has this J. Krishnamurti influence, which is a very free mind. He's not caught by the tradition. He's an authentic yogi.

Did you have a close relationship to Krishnamacharya?

I cannot say I had a close relationship with Krishnamacharya, though I had contact with him. He spoke to me several times to tell me things that he thought were important for me to hear. He told me that *viveka-khyati*—the dawning of deep discrimination between the real and the unreal, and one of the highest goals of yoga—is *Ishvara-khyati*. *Ishvara* means "God." *Khyati* means "dawning, awakening." He said the meaning of yoga is to recognize God in your life.

I felt a certain amount of fear, because Krishnamacharya had power. I felt awe and respect for the breadth of his knowledge and wisdom. Desikachar was studying the *Brahma Sutras*, which is this enormous text, with him. When Krishnamacharya was ready to start, Desikachar would say the first word of the last *sloka* they were on and the whole thing would come out by memory.

A friend of mine who went to see Desikachar in the early seventies was interested in astrology. Krishnamacharya was known as a great astrologer. Desikachar arranged a meeting for my friend with Krishnamacharya. Krishnamacharya saw a piece of paper with the birth date of my friend. He looked at the birth date, looked at my friend, and said, "Impossible." My friend thought he was crazy. Desikachar said, "My father is an unusual man. Maybe you should check." My friend called his mother in San Francisco. She called the hospital. The hospital did some research and found out that he was not born when he thought he was.

Why did you decide to become a teacher?

Between 1974 and 1978, I spent nearly three years in India with Desikachar. At a certain point, he said, "Go home." "What am I going to do?" I asked. He said, "Why don't you teach. You know too much. Why don't you go home and teach." I wasn't even thinking about being a yoga teacher before Desikachar encouraged me. I thought I might be a professor in religious studies. Sometimes I thought I would go to medical school. I wasn't clear. I was just studying yoga because I was fascinated.

What does your personal practice consist of?

My personal practice at this stage in my life is helping me understand who I am. What's my place? What's my work? It's what we call *dharma*. Deep self-reflection. Looking at who I really am and what I really want. I don't want to be overtaken by the momentum of busyness. I use my practice to keep checking into what I want to achieve before I am done with this life, what I want to accomplish for myself and for the world that I am in.

Do you put more emphasis on meditation than asana?

Pranayama, meditation, chanting, and prayer. I maintain my body and my health with *asana*. Occasionally, for fun, I challenge myself with *asana*.

Death is certain, although it's arrival is unknown. How do you cope with the uncertainty of death?

You use awareness of impermanence, of death, as a way of helping you appreciate the beauty of the present moment, and of helping you look deeply at what's important. You use that as motivation to reorganize your priorities and get to work. The teachings of the traditions say that death can happen at any moment. And when you die, it isn't over. What happens to you after you die can be very unpleasant, or pleasant, depending upon the *karma*, the momentum that you've created.

To people who think that they have forever I say, "Meditate on death." You only have a finite amount of time, and it's going to end very quickly. So get to work. It's not the great anxiety. It's the great appreciation for this moment to help you reorganize your priorities, so you can make intelligent choices.

And when we die?

I don't know. I know what the tradition says. The tradition says that you are swept up in the winds of your *karma*. So what you want to do is train your mind and purify your system. What can I say? There's more going on than we can perceive on a rational level.

Do you believe in the eternity of the soul?

I wouldn't say that I definitely believe. There's a distinction between faith and belief. I have deep faith in the teachings of these yogic traditions. It doesn't mean I have a cognitive clarity about what's going to happen. The rationale mind can't go beyond a certain point. I have faith that it's important for me to get to the root of the meaning of life. Death for me is a mirror of life. I use death meditation to make me alert, so I don't waste time.

When I was a kid I saw a cartoon. Bugs Bunny is in the desert. And there is this little teeny tent. Bugs Bunny sticks his head in the tent. It's a huge palace. He pulls his head out. His neck gets long and wraps around the tent. He puts his head in the tent again, and there is this enormous space. That's the practice of yoga. It takes me into the vastness in the core of my being.

Gary Kraftsow has taught yoga and practiced yoga therapy since 1976. At the age of nineteen, he traveled to Madras to meet T.K.V. Desikachar and his father, T. Krishnamacharya, initiating a link to the *Viniyoga* tradition that has become his life-long dedication. In 1983 he completed a Master's program in psychology and religion, focusing his study on health as a paradigm for spiritual transformation. Gary is an internationally known educator in the *Viniyoga* lineage, conducting retreats, trainings, and seminars throughout the United States and Europe. He is the only American to receive the *Viniyoga* Special Diploma, recognizing his ability to train teachers and therapists in this lineage. Gary continues his studies with T.K.V. Desikachar and lives on the island of Maui with his family.

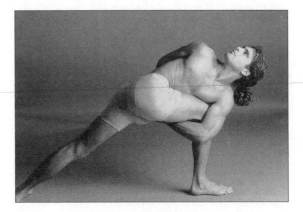

BRYAN KEST
LOS ANGELES

[This interview was conducted at a restaurant Bryan Kest opened below his yoga studio. Though the restaurant was still open, Kest was no longer the owner.]

Who would have guessed I would have opened this restaurant, and eight months later I would have it taken away. It's amazing. I lost every penny I had.

Not your life savings, but everything you invested?

It was my life savings.

It was a major lesson. Let go. Don't be attached. It's easy to walk away from $5,000 or $10,000. Try walking away from $100,000 that you spent the last umpteen years saving. I lost it all. I'm thankful. For one week, I can't tell how stressed out I was. Everything I ever worked for, everything I had in savings was all gone. Then I took a deep breath and said, "This is my lesson. This is what I've drawn in my life. This is what I need. Let it go. Trust." And that's what it did. I'm totally okay with it.

Most people who lost $100,000 here couldn't come back and eat. It would give them indigestion.

They all know I lost it. It was successful on one level. This restaurant has the potential to be really successful, so I feel like the vision was right, but it's not for me. More importantly, I lost a lot of money, which I needed to lose, in order to be okay with losing that much money. It really showed me how attached I was to it. There I was preaching non-attachment every moment and I was attached. I think the right lessons come to me when I need to have them.

That's what we work on in yoga. We get out of being the controller, the dictator. We breathe and we listen, and we're open to receive. Everything is an opportunity to learn and grow from. There are no mistakes. There is nothing bad. Everything that happens that doesn't sit well with you is a challenge to you to become okay with it, to breathe into it, and to not be so reactive to it. Some people never get it their whole life. They are fighting and resisting and controlling. And they die miserable and unhappy.

How did you discover yoga?

I was in the right place at the right time. I was on Maui in 1979 and David Williams had just come back from India. He is the second Westerner to study with K. Pattabhi Jois. He is the first person to bring *ashtanga* back to America and start teaching it. David started a class on Maui, and my dad got really into it. He told me to do yoga or to move out of the house. I picked yoga.

How old were you?

Fifteen.

Were you hooked?

The first six months I hated it. I was a football player and a meat-and-potatoes boy from Detroit. Stretching was the last thing that I enjoyed doing. I didn't see any benefit from it. It was very painful, but my dad forced me to do it. I didn't have a choice. One day I was mowing the lawn, and when I was done, I remember taking deep breaths from my head to my toes. I was vibrating. I was totally alive and I felt so good. Something inside me clicked. You just can't deny the truth of yoga.

Did you decide to teach at that point?

Teaching didn't come for years down the road, but I practiced yoga daily. I moved to California, and I worked as a busboy in a restaurant. One day, someone who knew I practiced yoga asked me to teach them. I said, "Okay." Someone else found out about it, and they asked me to teach them. I said, "Okay." Then someone else who owned a clinic for people with eating disorders—anorexia and bulimia—asked me if I would teach in the clinic. I started teaching yoga to these people. A lot of the clients were rich and influential. One owned a big health fitness center and asked me to teach there. It took a life of its own. If you told me I would have been a teacher, I would have said you were insane. It just evolved naturally.

Why did you travel to India?

I felt hypocritical, because I had never been to India. My yoga was valid. I knew what I was doing, but I wanted to feel where yoga came from. I wanted to feel the people. I wanted to taste it. I wanted to smell it. I saved up some money, bought a ticket to India, and spent a year studying yoga with Pattabhi Jois. I was twenty-five, so I had been teaching for about five years.

Was that transforming to your practice and to your life?

I learned more about yoga from being around the people in India. Yoga comes from the culture of India. The culture of India comes from yoga. Yoga takes on many shapes and forms. It's not just these physical movements. Yoga is a philosophy. There are different ways to practice yoga and one of the ways is *asana*. Most people in India do not practice *asana*.

When I went to India, I had all this muscle mass from when I used to lift weights. I couldn't lose the weight, because the yoga was so strong. But my muscles were preventing me from getting into some poses. I wanted to lose weight so badly. You have to be careful of what you ask for. Within a week I had hepatitis and 104° fever. I lost twenty pounds in seven days.

You could have lost your life.

I came very close to dying. They misdiagnosed me. My eyeballs turned brown. My urine turned brown. My skin turned yellow. I lay in bed for a month.

And after you recovered?

One day, I walked out of Pattabhi Jois' place. I felt so open and aware and sensitive. I thought, "Now what?" Someone said to me,

"You've got to try *Vipassana* meditation. It's amazing." It sounded so right. It sounded like the next step. I went up to northern India and I did it. It was a powerful experience that changed everything.

It was really amazing and highly transformative. That was the major transformative aspect of my trip to India as far as my spiritual practice goes. It gave me something beyond the physical practice.

Vipassana meditation is not easy. You meditate for twelve hours a day. You're not allowed to talk. You're not allowed to read. You're not allowed to write. You're not allowed to listen to music. But you get grounded in a meditation practice. You spend ten days honing the practice. It makes you look at yourself and deal with yourself, because there are no distractions. It's the hardest thing I've ever done in my entire life.

At some point did you think you weren't going to make it?

Oh, yeah! I wanted to run away so bad, but I've done nine of them since then. It's the most powerful thing I've ever done. I highly recommend it.

What has influenced your style of teaching?

I come from a highly competitive background. That's why I teach what I teach. We're all so competitive. We love to compete, but competition hinders our practice. Then we get judgmental and critical about ourselves. I try to empower people to let them know that they are already perfect. Yoga teaches that you are already enlightened. You've just got to wake up and realize it. The goal of yoga is *chit vrtti nirodhah*—the cessation of the fluctuations of the mind. It's quieting your mind down, not sticking your leg farther behind your head. Let's use our bodies as a tool to challenge our mind.

No matter how much yoga you do or bluegreen algae you chew, in a hundred years your physical body is not going to be here. Your body is limited. The unlimited aspect of who you are is your mind. If your practice doesn't move into your mind, then you're staying in the realm of limits and you have a very superficial practice. We have to bring our mind into our practice. The by-product of yoga is an amazingly resilient body, but it's not really about the body. It's about the mind. How can I use these poses to be more accepting of myself? How can I use these poses to practice being less reactive in difficult situations? How can I use these poses to get out of my ego and make it okay to take a break? The healthiest person isn't the person who goes the farthest in the pose. The healthiest person is a person whose mind is so quiet that they can listen to what their body is saying and honor it. Your body is talking to you. Are you listening? Or are you too busy trying to get somewhere?

Competing is about winning something or getting something. It's not about healing. They are different objectives. When you're competing, you end up pushing your body past where it wants to go in order to get to where you want to be, instead of listening to where your body wants to be and honoring it. I bet you can't think of one competition on the whole planet that's healthy for you. One time I said that to someone and they said, "Chess. What's so unhealthy about chess?" I said, "If you're attached to winning, you're competing. And if you're not winning, I bet you build up a lot of stress."

Stress manifests tension in your body, which blocks the flow of energy moving through your body. Stress is a breeding ground for disease and discomfort. The root of all disease on the planet is blockage of energy. What blocks energy more than tense knots in your body, or dead dormant spots that never get awakened? We use the poses to awaken the body. We don't use the poses to make you loose. Flexibility is a by-product. The goal is aliveness. You don't have to be loose to be alive. We use the poses to create friction all over the body. The body sends blood, which flushes out toxicity and creates aliveness. In the process, you create awareness. The first step to healing is awareness. Once you're aware of something then you can work on it.

Do you still enjoy competition?

Well, that depends on what your definition of competition is. I'm not attached to the outcome anymore. If I'm competing for the fun of it, maybe, and is that really competition? Yoga teaches non-competition. It's a non-competitive endeavor.

What is your philosophy behind the donation box?

First of all, I want to make yoga available to everybody. I don't want it to be about money. Money is not the priority. That's part of the problem with society right now. Secondly, it's my own yoga to trust in the universe and not be so controlling. I don't have someone sit outside of class and collect the money. If I'm supposed to make money, I will. If I'm not, I won't.

In class you say, "It's about feeling good, not just looking good." Please elaborate.

There are five billion people in this world. That means there should be five billion different ways to look. I see a lot of people making themselves sick trying to jam their body into some stereotypical way that society has brainwashed them into thinking they should look. I see men and women getting implants. I see exercise taking this perverted detour. The original intention of exercise was to heal and to maintain health. Now I see it as having nothing to do with health. I see most exercises based on looking good. They actually make you less healthy. You overdevelop the obvious muscles. You take drugs to enhance that. You ignore the rest, and you become more out of balance.

If you feel good, don't you think you should look good? If you don't like the way you look when you feel good, then you should reassess the way you think you should look. We're all so stuck on looking good. I understand the objective. I want to look good. But let's do it with awareness. Let's not base our opinion of ourselves on what other people think about us. Have you ever read a statistic that says prettier people are healthier or happier? If your self-esteem and self-value is based on how you look, then you're in trouble. I guarantee you one thing—no matter how pretty you are, it will change. When it changes, what are you going to do and who are you?

How does one overcome the attachment to physical appearance?

Overcoming it is not easy, but seeing through it is a little easier. Once you understand that, you will slowly start to overcome it. The first step in any healing program is awareness. You can't heal anything you are not aware of. I still deal with it. I teach it every day, and I still catch myself being judgmental or critical about myself. It's a lifetime's work, but the less judgmental I am the better I feel every day.

The goal of everybody's life is peace. Everybody is running around like a little ant trying to do what they think they have to do in order to get peace. I look at peace as a state of being, not something that you can get on the outside. If you base your happiness on getting somewhere, when you get there you're just going to want something else, because that's your mentality. "I'll be happy when…"

The root of being happy is self-acceptance. My happiness does not depend on anything that's happening on the outside. Whatever is happening on the outside will change. It's out of my control. If my happiness is based on something that's out of my control, I'm setting myself up for disappointment and frustration. My happiness has to be based on something inside that transcends all my experiences.

Even though it's futile, it seems easier and more seductive to search for peace and happiness outside ourselves.

We have to realize it's not easier. It's just what we were taught. It's a false teaching. It's temporary gratification. You cannot control the things that are happening around you. You are not in control. There is only one thing in your life that you are in control of, and that is your intention or your volition. That's it. Everything else can be taken away from you. If your happiness depends on something else, you set yourself up for frustration and disappointment because that can be taken away. Your happiness should be dependent on something that will always be there and that you can control. Your happiness should not be dependent on anything on the outside. This way no one can take your happiness away from you. You're at peace. That's self-acceptance.

Yoga class is the greatest environment to work on self-acceptance. The number one attachment any human being has is their body. When you do yoga a lot of stuff comes up—judgment, criticism, frustration, competitiveness. It becomes this amazing place to work on letting go of that stuff. It's a safe, forgiving environment to see yourself and to let it go. "I'm being judgmental." Smile and let it go. "I'm being critical." Smile and let it go. "I'm trying hard to get somewhere, instead of making it okay for me to be here." Smile and let it go. Eventually the things that you work on in yoga class will start transcending yoga class—like being less reactive in a difficult situation. The next time someone flips you off, you won't be so reactive. You won't build tension in your body and poison yourself.

What is the importance of yoga and meditation?

Yoga and meditation are the most optimal situations for me to learn and grow, and become more connected with my spirituality and the universe. Yoga and meditation are the optimal situations for healing. There is nothing more practical you could ever do than yoga. Yoga keeps you alive. It keeps you supple. On the physical level, there is nothing more important than suppleness. Suppleness represents healthy, vibrant, toned muscles that are relaxed enough to let your skeleton fall into place. When your skeleton falls into place, you experience alignment. When you are aligned, all the energy moves freely, and you feel light and good. Forget about all the spiritual mumbo jumbo. That's just physical, practical stuff. You can't beat it. There is nothing more appropriate than yoga.

Does yoga and meditation help you stay in the present moment?

That's the goal. Fear and anger come from things that happened to you. Anxiety and apprehension come from things that are going to happen to you. In the moment, there's only purity. The goal of meditation is to make you more present. Everything that has happened to us is influencing our experience right now. It's hard to have a childlike newness to every situation. Yoga on a physical level moves you through your body and helps release all the stuff you're holding onto in the form of knots and tension. When you finish, you feel lighter and more present. It teaches us how to release what we're holding and how not to accumulate more. If we don't accumulate more, the next time we do yoga we can go deeper.

Did yoga have an impact on your diet?

I was your average American guy who grew up on meat and potatoes. I lived on Twinkies and Hostess cupcakes. Rarely ate salad. Then I became a total vegetarian. I was even a strict macrobiotic for a while. Yoga was a part of that. I have come back to eating meat, but the difference is I have come back to it with consciousness.

The other day I craved a soft drink. I gave myself a soft drink. When I drank it, I was aware that I was drinking a soft drink. I was aware there was nothing alive in it, and I shouldn't do it that often.

But did you enjoy it?

I totally enjoyed it! It tasted good! But I did it with awareness. I have come full circle. I'm almost back to where I was eating when I was a kid, minus the junk food. I don't overdo it with the meat.

Is moderation the key?

Not only moderation, but also consciousness. I'm not blindly doing these things because that's what I grew up doing. I know the ramifications of what I'm doing, and I chose to do it.

Some would say you have to be a vegetarian to be following a yogic path.

Some would say you don't.

Some people can wake up, eat bacon and eggs, and feel great. Some people like to have fruit in the morning. Some people don't like to eat anything in the morning. Who's right and who's wrong? None of them are right or wrong. I envy the people who can eat bacon and eggs for breakfast. I miss it!

I look at the body as a separate entity. Our job is to learn how to have a healthy relationship with it. If you treated your best friend, your siblings, your spouse, or your parents with the kind of judgment, criticism, frustration, and expectations that you treat yourself, they wouldn't stay in your life very long. No one wants to be judged. No one wants to be criticized. No one wants expectations of always having to work so hard to get somewhere, yet that's the way most people treat themselves. Yoga practice is learning how to have a healthy relationship with your body. Instead of telling your body what to do, ask it what it wants to do. Then listen to what it says. Let your body tell you what it wants. It knows what it wants.

Every day you practice yoga, you're different. You get into the poses, and your body starts to let you know where it's at today. Your body has moods, just like your mind has moods. If you're in a quiet, meditative mood, you don't go to a party. That would be counterproductive. If your body is in the mood for working gently, you don't push hard. If your body has a lot of energy and is in the mood for working hard, then you should work hard. You listen and find out where you're at, and work with it. When you start listening to your body, and being more accepting of your body, and less judgmental and critical of your body, your relationships with other people will change. You will stop being judgmental of other people. You will stop being critical of other people.

The most amazing quality that anybody can have is the quality of listening. You can become a good listener by listening to yourself in your yoga practice. Your body knows exactly what it needs for balance. The question is are you listening?

Everybody on this planet is a channel. We have something to offer. Most of us are not connected to what we're channeling, because our minds are clogged with so much thinking and so much dogma and so much busyness. Your body is one big antenna for truth. If you get really quiet and really listen, then you can start becoming that channel. You open your body up, and it becomes a receiver. You can offer what you're receiving to the planet. Our greatest mission is to be able to help someone. We learn how to do it by helping ourselves.

Our culture says you are a very selfish person when you focus on helping yourself.

I disagree. We're misinterpreting the word selfish. I don't think you have anything to give anybody until you give to yourself. It's not selfish. If you want me to contribute, I have to have something to contribute. Give me some time to go cultivate it. If you don't feed yourself, you will die. Yoga is our time to feed ourselves. That's where we replenish, so we have more to give others. How are you supposed to heal anybody else, if you don't know how to heal yourself? How are we supposed to heal this planet, if we don't know how to heal ourselves?

If you eliminated your personal practice do you think you could continue to be a channel?

Not at all. When I stop doing yoga for whatever reason, my teaching totally suffers. I lose my connection to what I am doing. Mostly I lose my connection to myself. One good thing about a meditation practice or a yoga practice is that you take time every day to connect to yourself. When I practice, I come from a place of connection. When I am connected to myself, I am connected to everybody else. The longer you go not connecting yourself, the less you come from that place. And pretty soon, you are not connected at all.

Bryan Kest has been practicing yoga for over eighteen
years, starting at the age of fifteen in Hawaii with David
Williams, the first person to bring *Ashtanga* yoga to Ameri-
ca. He spent over a year studying intensively with K. Pattabhi
Jois, Sanskrit scholar and *Ashtanga* yoga master, in Mysore,
India. Bryan studied holistic health and nutrition at Ryokan
College, and was a yoga therapist on staff at Esteem, a Santa
Monica treatment center for people with eating disorders.
He has been teaching for thirteen years and is the owner of
the Santa Monica Power Yoga Center. His unique teaching
style has been popularized by his three-part video series
Bryan Kest's Power Yoga.

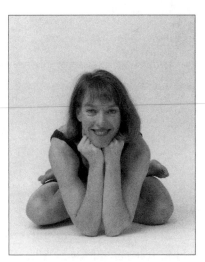

JULIE LAWRENCE
PORTLAND

How did you discover yoga?

I began yoga at a very difficult time in my life. I was twenty-one years old, and I had just gotten married. My husband, Bruce, was killed in Vietnam. I went to live with his family in southern California for three months. It was a completely new setting. One of his mother's friends said, "Why don't you and Julie go to a yoga class with me?" We really couldn't have cared less, but we went. We even drove through Los Angeles rush hour traffic to get there.

The yoga class made me feel better. I couldn't articulate what it was about this yoga class that made a difference, but it made a difference, so I continued to go.

When Bruce was killed, I moved away from the church that I

had been going to. Yoga wasn't a religious experience in that sense, but there was a sense of connectedness. There was a sense of peace. I still couldn't articulate it. All I knew was that this felt good.

When you left the church, did you feel like you couldn't trust God anymore?

That's exactly why I left the church. I felt betrayed. I was angry. I was in pain. Bruce and I had been together about four years. One of our first dates was the senior prom. We dated all through college. We got engaged and decided that if he had to go to Vietnam, we would not get married. When he got orders to go to Vietnam, he said he wanted to get married. I said, "Let's do it." We were together for a month before he went. That was in October, and he was there until August. He was due to come home in sixty days when he was killed.

It was really hard. I was only twenty-one, and I had my life cut out from under me. Since I didn't have a lot of internal strength, I fell apart. Taking those yoga classes was the first step in bringing me back to health.

Did you ever return to the church?

I gave it up when Bruce was killed. I definitely have come back to a sense of the Universe, Energy, God, or Goddess. It's very present in my life, but I don't label it necessarily one thing or another.

How has your life experience allowed you to offer solace to others who are in pain?

One of the ways that I can help people in a similar situation is by sharing my pain with them—to let them know that I experienced the pain of losing someone and that the yoga helped me.

Now, albeit many years later, I'm happy and I'm healthy. That's the unspoken part of what I want to say—it will change. I feel a very important part of that change was the process of yoga. I don't believe in preaching to people. We touch people most deeply by being who we are.

I teach week-long retreats, and I can talk about practice, but if they see me in the yoga room at six o'clock in the morning doing my practice before I teach all day, that has a much stronger impact than my yapping to them about practice. When someone is in pain, if I can share my pain, and they can see that I have been able to pull myself back together again, I think that speaks for itself.

Out of my greatest tragedy came my life's work, my life's inspiration. Out of the mud comes the lotus.

Does the pain ever go away?

It changes with time, but it's always there. I am still in contact with Bruce's family and that gives me great joy. I think it gives them joy, too.

Two months after discovering yoga, I went to Europe for a year. Yoga was something I could do in my hotel room, in a youth hostel, or wherever. Yoga was a constant. It was something that I could return to amidst the emotional chaos of traveling to a new country every three or four weeks. It was something that, even then, I realized came from within me. That was a first for me. I feel our society doesn't support or value our being self-reliant in a deep, inner way.

I was brought up in Berkeley, but I led what I would call a sheltered life. Becoming a widow at age twenty-one and then going to Europe virtually on my own for a year were both huge stretches. The trip taught me self-reliance.

Were you traveling solo?

I was traveling solo some of the time. I would meet people in the youth hostels, and we would travel together. I did go from the United States with a girlfriend, but she went on her own shortly after we arrived there. I thought that we were going to travel together, but we ended up going our separate ways.

I was a scared and lost soul who was searching. I put myself in a lot of new situations. Traveling by myself on trains, not speaking the language, and dealing with men were difficult in foreign countries. I visited relatives with whom I really couldn't converse, because they didn't speak English and I didn't speak Italian. We spoke fractured French. That was fun, but it was still scary. Throughout all the external stimulation that was going on, with all that I was seeing and all that I was doing, I could go back home to my hotel room and do my yoga and there was a sense of continuity.

Did you have a meditation practice in Europe?

I did not.

You were strictly practicing asana?

Right. But through the accessibility of the body, I was able to become quiet within myself. It wasn't anything that I was aware of at the time, but I believe it was transforming me even then. It was transforming me in terms of helping me deal with my emotional pain. It gave me solace. It gave me a sense of peace that comes through grace.

Also, it taught me to trust. My mother was over-protective of me. She taught me to never trust strangers. When I was a child, a young girl who was seven was kidnapped in Berkeley. It was in all the papers, and I got very scared by it. I think that really impressed upon me that you don't trust anybody. Yoga has taught me to trust and to open my heart. Some of that is through the physical practice.

I was scared of meditation, because I felt that if I went inside there probably wasn't anything there. Just a void. I felt very uncomfortable with the idea of going inside and really getting to know myself. I think that comes from a basic lack of self-esteem as a child. But yoga is transformative in a core way. It's doing its work without me making it happen. That's what I really like about teaching—watching people light up. Watching people feel an "ah-ha," even though they may not understand exactly where that's going to take them.

How did you overcome your fear and develop a meditation practice?

The physical practice led me to the need for deepening. The practice led me to want it. It wasn't something that I thought I should do. Instead, it was something that I yearned for. What I was yearning for was that sense of connection and trusting, that connection to something greater than myself.

I started to meditate, and then I took a step back and started to do *pranayama*. After I started doing *pranayama*, the meditation was a lot easier. I really had the monkey mind. It was very hard for me to meditate until I started practicing *pranayama*. I learned to quiet my mind much more through the breathing, then the meditation could come. Iyengar says that you don't have a *pranayama* practice unless it's a daily practice. That is a pretty strict guideline. I did that, and I have been doing that. The fruit of *pranayama* is meditation.

How did your yoga practice develop when you returned to the states?

When I came home, I moved to Oregon. I did yoga with Lilias Folan on TV, then I finally found a teacher in Portland. She introduced me to Iyengar yoga and to Judith Lasater. I took classes in

Portland continually for another four years. In 1977, I went to the Feathered Pipe Ranch for a workshop with Judith, and I was hooked. It's a wonderfully beautiful place, and a very supportive, loving environment. The hills, the lake, and the woods keep you grounded. This year was my twentieth anniversary of going to Feathered Pipe, and they asked me to teach.

Shortly after my first trip to Feathered Pipe, I started teaching yoga in Portland. Teaching was not something I aspired to do. Someone said to me, "I'm going away for the summer. Would you like to teach my class?" I said, "No." He said, "Well, would you help me teach the last class?" I said, "Sure." The experience wasn't something I anticipated. It was wonderful. It was connecting with people in a way I didn't imagine. I taught his class for the summer, and in the fall I began to teach my own classes. My first class was six people, mostly friends. My yoga practice, and certainly my teaching, has been a very organic process. They have flowered in their own time. Yoga has taught me that everything happens in its own time. I'm beginning to trust that.

What else have you learned from yoga?

In 1978, I decided I to go to Pune to study with Iyengar. That's when I got very serious about daily practice. I didn't have a teacher at the time. I discovered that although I didn't have a teacher, I could learn an enormous amount through trusting my practice, through just going to the mat and doing yoga. That was a big "ah-ha." The practice really taught me that I could learn from my own internal wisdom. As long as I was doing yoga with my mind involved and focused, I learned a tremendous amount. If I was thinking about the shopping list, it didn't happen. But if I focused my mind, if I really concentrated on what was going on at the moment I was practicing, I learned a tremendous amount.

Were you excited about your upcoming trip?

I was terrified.

Had you met Iyengar?

No.

But you were doing Iyengar yoga?

I was doing Iyengar yoga.

What was your motivation for going to India?

I wanted to go to the source. I wanted to *do* it. It was a stretch for me. I was fairly new in the world of Iyengar yoga. I had heard he was a tough master. He and I hit it off really well. He was gruff with me, but he would have a twinkle in his eye. I found myself many times just laughing out loud, and he got that. I knew he was being hard on me, and the harshness didn't matter. The teaching came through. I went back the very next year, which was a bit too soon. I didn't have time to integrate everything I had learned the first year.

What did you think you learned from India that you would not have learned without that experience?

That's a very interesting question. I understand yoga better, because I have been to the place of its roots. I have seen Iyengar in his culture. He's very strict, but when I see him in the milieu of his life, his strictness makes more sense to me. Also, it was important to see the way the Iyengars live and to see their dedication to what they do. Their house is built twenty feet away from the yoga center, and they go back and forth. They live this. They eat, sleep, and practice yoga twenty-four hours a day. That commitment has been important for me to see. It has deepened my own commitment.

Sometimes I feel that I don't have a life outside of yoga. It even takes up my evenings. The people that I see generally are yoga people. The food that I eat now has changed because I have done yoga for so many years. It's all-encompassing. I saw that aspect most deeply when I saw the way the Iyengars live. Geeta cooks the food for the family. She teaches public classes. She was running a women's intensive, overseeing poses that they are going to use in a CD-ROM, and helping to compile her father's collected works. This woman's commitment is unbelievable.

The way people live their lives is a very important model. We learn a lot regardless of the way they live. We either learn what to do or what not to do. Seeing Geeta's dedication has deepened my commitment.

Is their yoga center in an area of poverty?

No. It is in a nice residential area. One of the wonderful things is that when you are visiting them, you stay in a hotel in the community, rather than live at the institute. Students walk the streets or bike to get there. We partake of the community, whether it's the smog, the traffic, or the beautiful fruit stalls. We see the people who are living on the streets. We walk through that to get to this nicer, green, residential area.

One of the things that I have learned is that just because these people are living in a way that is different from my own, it doesn't mean they are unhappy. They have their sense of community. They have their loved ones. They have a life that is very different from mine, but I'm not to judge that.

How far is the center from your hotel?

It's about a twenty-five minute walk each way, and that's really nice. After a good yoga class, what I usually want to do is walk.

How much have you assimilated?

I feel less like an outsider now than I used to. When I first started going to India, which was seventeen years ago, people would turn and stare. They don't do that as much, because there are more Westerners.

Pune is a hill town about five hours outside of Bombay. It's not in the boonies, but it is its own place. Pune is a university town that's enjoying a surge of prosperity because it's also a computer center. There are a lot of computer engineers in Pune, so it's more connected to the world. There is more acceptance of foreigners. I don't think I will ever feel totally assimilated. I'm only there for a month at a time, and I don't speak the language.

Describe a typical day in Pune.

A normal day would be to awaken, do *pranayama* in my room, do my personal practices, have some tea, and then walk to the Institute for class, which is generally from nine to noon. We would break, go have lunch with a group of people that were taking the class, come back at four, do some restoratives, and have *pranayama* class. I usually stay and observe one of the evening classes, go have dinner, then go back to the hotel room, read, and fall asleep.

Does Geeta focus on yoga for women?

It's not limited to that, but she did a women's intensive in January this year. I joined together with sixty other women from sixteen countries to attend this first time ever event. Geeta said our models have been male and there are some ways in which women need to practice yoga differently. We have to take care of our bodies. We push too hard. There was great permission in that for me—to honor what my body needs. Women's cycles are more concrete than men's cycles. There are times in the cycle when you don't feel like working as hard. She has taught me to honor and to trust my own body more.

How has your trust developed?

In the beginning I was trusting people, trusting my body, and trusting the yoga process to take me where I needed to go. Right now it's about trusting my meditation practice. If I sit and I get a very clear message to go do something, I do it.

When we follow our inner voice, we learn what connection, community, synchronicity, and God are all about. It's the mystery. We can't know the mystery, but that's where the energy lies. If we can trust the mystery, that's the piece that can transform us, because it's the unknown. It's the part that we have to venture into. Living our lives on automatic and staying stuck in our habits can be a sort of personal death. The opposite of that is the mystery, moving into the unknown. Courting the mystery makes me feel vital. I can't understand it, I can't explain it, but I can feel it.

Fear is very real. We have to face our fears, because our fears are the obstacles. Fear is in our mind. Our mind creates these fanciful things that are worse than reality. It is only by acknowledging, confronting, and dealing with our fears that we are going to get beyond them to whatever is next.

One of the important lessons of yoga is concentration—to notice when the mind is spinning out on the fear and to bring it back to the present moment, the direct experience.

What was your motivation for opening your own yoga center?

I always said I didn't want a center, because I didn't want to manage people. When my husband, Michael, and I got together, I was teaching at various sites around town. He encouraged me to bring it all together in one place. So I found a space, and I was the only teacher for a while. Now there are five of us, and we have twenty-three classes a week. I've had to learn things about managing, like the balance between encouraging them to have input, and that I'm the one who pays the rent. The ideas that come out of our time together are usually better than the ideas that I come up with alone. It's my yoga center, but I enjoy encouraging them to shine, so that it's not just my show. I don't want it to be my show.

Is your husband a member of the yoga community?

He takes classes. He's a runner, so he spends more time beating the pavement than doing yoga. He realizes that the yoga helps balance his life. He has been a very important part of the growth of my yoga practice, and certainly my yoga business. He is extremely supportive emotionally.

Is it difficult to maintain and honor your own personal practice with the demands of running a yoga center?

Always. There are many things that can eat it up. Rodney Yee once told me that he practiced in his hallway with his kids climbing all over him. That's a little gem as far as I'm concerned. He's a beautiful practitioner of yoga. If this man practices in the hallway with kids climbing all over him, what are my excuses?

Sometimes I practice just for me, and sometimes I practice for my teaching. My tendency is to practice for my teaching. I need to remind myself that yoga practice is a privilege and that I deserve to practice only for me once in a while. To practice what I need to work on, or what I'm working towards, is delicious.

What is the purpose of yoga practice?

Yoga training is about seeing reality clearly. It's about awareness. Life is never going to be exactly what we want it to be. It's about how we choose to react. It's making a choice to respond differently. Anytime something really irritates and aggravates us, we are just as hooked in as we were before we ever did yoga. In not liking something, you are just as attached to it as if you desired it.

So the practice should give insight into life?

It has to. Otherwise, we're just going through the motions. It has to be relevant. That's what keeps us all going.

How has yoga transformed your life?

Yoga has made me friends with myself. I didn't like myself before I started yoga, because I didn't know myself. Yoga has brought me a sense of self-confidence and self-worth. That comes directly from some of the physical work, which brings a sense of inner strength.

I have never come away from a yoga practice feeling less than when I began. I am always more than. I always feel better. That's what I want to inspire in my students.

Yoga is about feeling more alive. Yoga does that for me on so many levels.

Julie Lawrence has been practicing yoga for thirty years and has been teaching throughout the United States and internationally for twenty-two years. She has studied in India many times with internationally acclaimed yoga teacher B.K.S. Iyengar and his daughter, Geeta, and has served on the board of the Iyengar Yoga National Association of the United States. Julie has appeared on numerous radio and television programs and is the creator of *Yoga for Health and Relaxation* audiotapes. Her unique presentation integrates the Eastern practice of yoga with the Western lifestyle. Julie enjoys gardening at her home in the Pacific Northwest.

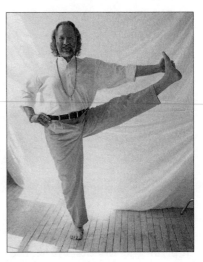

ALAN FINGER
NEW YORK CITY

Paramahansa Yogananda, one of the world's most recognized and influential yogis, introduced your father, Mani Finger, to yoga. How did this transpire?

My father was shell-shocked when a bomb went off in the Second World War in North Africa where he was with the Royal Army. He got involved in drugs because his nerves were shot. That's how I grew up the first eight years of my life in South Africa.

Then my father went to America on a business trip to a big convention in Los Angeles. Yogananda happened to be giving a lecture at the Ambassador Hotel where my father was staying. Someone who he was with said, "There's a yoga guy with long hair and robes. Let's go see what it's about." My father would have rather gone drinking, but he went. Afterwards, he went up to Yogananda and bowed down to him. Yogananda said, "You are very troubled. I will teach you *kriya* yoga. You will become a yogi and all of your children will follow." And that's what my father did. He learned *kriya* yoga with Yogananda, went to India and studied with Sivananda, came back to South Africa, and started teaching.

This chance encounter with Yogananda transformed your father.

Exactly. He had a back injury, and that back injury has plagued him on and off his whole life. A long time ago, his doctor performed surgery to try to rectify where the bones were shattered. Even still if they did the operation today, it's not something that's easily done. So he has had very weak legs since then, but overcame his weakness and dedicated himself to yoga.

How did you process your father's immersion into yoga?

Well, it was very slow. By the time I was fifteen, I was haunted by the past and by insecurities, because I did not have a balanced, stable family life until I was eight. I weighed 265 pounds by the time I was fifteen. I was seeing a psychiatrist and trying to get myself together. I was totally turned off, because the guy was fidgety and wasn't present. I went back and said to my father, "I've got psychosomatic problems, I've got these physical manifestations, but this guy's problems are worse than mine. I don't think he can help me. Can't you teach me through yoga how to cure my emotional problems and weight problem?"

He said, "Well, it's hard, my son. This is what you've got to do. When I wake up at four-thirty in the morning, you've got to wake up, too. You've got to meditate with me and do yoga postures." And that was about a three-hour process. "You've got to do it every day.

I'm not going to nag you. I'm not going to beg you. All I'm going to do is switch your light on at four-thirty. I will do that two or three times. It's up to you." I said, "I've got to do something. I'll try it."

Meditation and yoga practice wasn't easy, but within two weeks, I was starting to see results. In two months and three weeks I had lost 100 pounds, my energy changed, I felt in control of myself, and I started teaching yoga. The weight loss was from the *asanas* and from the discipline—being able to say, "This is what I'm going to eat and that's it."

Food was your drug of choice?

Food has always been where I would go to get my comfort. I realized it then. I have it under tremendous control, but I definitely have to keep watching the weight. Otherwise, I would be a big Buddha-type yogi.

Describe your morning practice with your father.

At four-thirty I would get up, wash my face and do *neti*—saltwater through the nose to clean the sinuses. Then I would go downstairs and do *kapala-bhati*, the purification breath, up to 1,008 times. Next I would sit down and do *pranayama* and meditation for about an hour-and-a-quarter. So *neti, kapala-bhati, pranayama,* and meditation took about an hour-and-a-half. Then my father and I would have lemon juice, honey, and water. We would do *asana* for another hour-and-a-half. Father was really into holding poses a long time. That was my practice, and I did it about three years.

When did you become a full-time yoga teacher?

When I was nineteen, my father had to have an operation on

his back, so I took over most of his classes and became a full-time yogi. He would give talks and teach a few classes. I stayed in South Africa until I was twenty-six. I got married, and we came to America because my first wife had met a lot of Americans when she was abroad and wanted to go to the states. I said, "All right, let's go." My brother was an American citizen through marriage, so it was easy for us to get in. We went to Washington, D.C. and opened up a yoga studio just outside of Columbia, Maryland.

I loved what I was doing, until my son got brain seizures from high temperature. I was driving in the snow at night taking him to the hospital. I couldn't handle the cold. I said, "I'm going to go to California." After my son recovered, we packed up and went to Los Angeles. I started two yoga studios—first, Yoga Tantra Institute and then, Yoga Works with Maty Ezraty.

After twelve years there, I felt it was time for a change. I came to New York and started Yoga Zone. The cold was pretty tough here, too. I thought, "Maybe I should go to Florida and try that." I was going to go, but my son said, "Dad, you really shouldn't go. You've built up here again, now you're going to go again. I'll help you. You need to make a real business and get all these yoga studios going. Go for it. Try another couple of years." I said, "Okay." It went like lightning. It built up very, very quickly.

What is Ishta *yoga?*

My father and I developed *Ishta* yoga. He started before me but didn't call it *Ishta*. Because yoga practices are so vast, I felt it was necessary to systemize yoga for Westerners, so they could get a better grasp. I wanted to present the essence of yoga. The normal tradition of teaching is through *shaktipat*, through a person sitting with their teacher and learning. Picking up the vibe. That's actually how I learned.

We said, "What can we call our style of yoga?" Father said, "Well, our system has always been very personal. It's about taking a person, watching for their weaknesses, guiding them through their weaknesses, and finding their right *sadhana*." Your *sadhana*, your practice, would be different in some ways than another person's, because we're all unique. I like the word *Ishta*, because it means "personal calling" or "your own soul's calling." It comes from *Ishta-devata*.

Why did you choose the name Yoga Zone?

I came up with that name because yoga puts us in a different zone. When you get into that zone, you're in a different place. Getting into that zone is what heals and rejuvenates. Not merely sweat. The real focus of *asana* is to release the blockages that intimidate and inhibit us, and to strengthen the muscles so we can sit comfortably to meditate for a long period of time without discomfort or falling to sleep.

What does your practice consist of today?

Now my practice varies. I practice a minimum of an hour on a rush day. I usually practice an hour-and-a-half to two hours. On weekends I can go three or four hours—an hour of meditation and *pranayama*, then two or three hours of yoga. I vary the *asanas* due to the time of year, whether it's hot, cold, or due to the energy at the time in the environment. I work out a routine, and that's the routine we teach for a couple of weeks in the studio. Sometimes it's hard, sometimes more gentle. Sometimes more heat generating, sometimes more cooling.

Why do you start with meditation?

I start with meditation for two reasons. First, it's best for me to meditate early in the morning before the hustle and the vibe of the city starts. Secondly, *asanas* develop a lot of heat in your system, and that heat needs to cool down before you start meditation. Otherwise, the energy can move in the wrong channels internally when you meditate. It's better to do *pranayama* and meditation, and then come into *asana* afterwards. It's very untraditional in that usually people do *asana*, take a break, do *pranayama*, take a break, and then meditate. If one has the time, this is the correct way to practice.

A lot of the *asana* people don't meditate. That's crazy. It's very easy to get caught in *asana* and trapped in the body, becoming more and more supple. That really is a loss to the real goal. The real goal is to be able to sit and meditate. Sit still. One is doing all these asanas to remove locks and inhibitions, so you can actually sit still and move into your divine path. Then yoga is complete. I find that a lot of schools don't really have a good balance between those two. Some do very sloppy yoga and meditate a lot. Others do very strong postures and don't meditate. Somewhere in the middle is the balance of everything, and that's what I'm striving to keep.

The *asanas* are not done to create an instant enlightened state. They're done to slowly realign the body—to strengthen muscles and clear energy channels so that you can channel energy in your system. That's the real purpose—to allow you ultimately to sit still. It's the cumulative work of the *asanas* and *pranayama* that changes the way the subtle body functions, and ultimately allows one to get into a state of meditation.

What is the value of meditation?

It puts me in touch with the divine part of my being, which is only attainable when the mind is completely still. To reach into Self-realization and God-realization you have to reach a state of complete stillness. Going into that place is what really fuels my system with *ananda*, bliss consciousness. That is the effervescence of the soul, which feeds the intellect of our body, the intellectual *chi*. Going into a state of nothing and allowing the brain waves to become quiet allows the soul to send out its signal. A meditative state is the best form of antioxidants that one could get.

You begin to see all of these things happen when you get into a state of nothingness. A state of nothingness is a state where there is no fragmentation in consciousness. It's where consciousness is complete, and when it's complete, it's genius. For me, not to go into that state is impossible, because I just don't feel right. I'm not inspired. If I don't meditate, the vibe, the power, the electricity, the peace, the effervescence does not come through. So, I have no option but to do it. I cannot go without meditation because I know it is my fuel and my reality. When you have tasted that and have been in the depth of clarity and stillness, to not have it just doesn't make sense. It's crazy. It's like saying, "I'm not going to breathe." You can't. In the thirty-six years I've been meditating, I have missed five days of practice. I don't do it because I care about what other people think or because I am a yogi. I do not feel the same. So, to me, it's obvious. To sit there and saturate myself in that state of consciousness is the major key to my existence. That's why I'm here.

Your soul radiates an energy, which is called bliss. That radiance of your soul is bliss in its experience, and it is divine intelligence, divine wisdom. You cannot get inspiration from your thinking. That's not inspiration, that's learning. If you are trying to feel inspired, you can't. It comes from the seed and works itself out.

Learning to get in touch and saturate yourself in that divine part is what inspires you in your whole life. Scientific tests have found that when people cry, the tears of joy and the tears of sadness have a different chemical make-up. One's acidic, one's alkaline. We're very interconnected. What's going on in your mind is going to effect your body. It's going to make it alkaline or acid. Alkaline if you're in peace.

Cleaning the mind affects every aspect of your life. When you meditate, you go into deep peace. The intelligence of peace comes through and your system heals itself. You become inspired. You achieve *viveka*, the ability to see things as they really are. You make choices that are correct. When you look through the windshield of your mind and it's muddy, a tree can look like the road. But if you clean the windshield, the way is obvious.

Is meditation a form of prayer?

Prayer is a process to surrender. You can pray, but you really don't have to surrender. If prayer leads one to total surrender and oneness, it is meditation. Meditation is an after-product of having surrendered.

Praying doesn't really have a big importance without self-study. Self-study has a huge importance—self-study with a small s, and then self-study with a big S. Self-study is much more important than prayer. Through self-study we achieve *tapas*, burning out the impurities of our behavioral practices, and *ishvara-pranidhana*, surrender to the universe. Prayer, unfortunately, is confusing to many people. It has all the visuals of how to reach God, but it doesn't really take you there unless you can totally surrender. Total surrender is very hard because the mind has a conscious aspect and an unconscious aspect, and we are not conscious of the unconscious aspect.

A parrot can say, "Good morning! How are you? Pretty parrot!" But grab that parrot by the neck. It doesn't say, "Let me go!" It squawks and goes back to its unconscious nature. And that is exactly the difference between prayer and meditation. In prayer, someone can say, "Brother, peace, and love." But the unconscious person underneath can financially cheat others, then go back to the church, donate some money, and it appears everything's okay. The true unconscious of the person is like the parrot squawking. You must reach into the unconscious mind by meditation and see what is really at the core of your being, and release the stuff that truly inhibits you. You must clean the unconscious mind by meditating.

When you meditate you stop the mind and see your unconscious. That's why meditation is not always nice for the beginner. It's tough, because you sit down and suddenly you see your behavioral patterns. But if you don't create stillness, you don't have a chance to see what ghosts are inside of you and release them.

So meditation can be a painful process.

It can be painful. Everyone needs a teacher to guide them through. All of us need direction to go into the darkness and look for the light. It's hard without a teacher. To go into the realms of the unknown, we need someone watching. Otherwise, we will touch on pain and then say, "Meditation's not for me, I'm a hatha yogi." Or, "I want to chant. The group energy is much more powerful to me." We don't want to look at the ghosts and see what's really there. But ultimately, everyone has to face the issues that haunt them and have been suppressed into the unconscious mind, and release them to achieve enlightenment.

Do you find teaching to be a great learning experience?

Teaching is a great learning experience, but so is doing. My own practice is where I find things and feel things within myself, and then communicate it to others.

When I had been practicing yoga for about a year, a series of events conspired to keep me in New York City longer than I intended, so I attended a weekend lecture you were giving at Yoga Zone. You led a meditation and I felt myself going to a deeper level than I had ever experienced before. Please explain this phenomenon.

There is an element of *shaktipat*, which means that the vibration of the teacher will draw and pull the student with them until they reach the same level of meditation. It's always nice to be in the presence of a teacher. If we sat now, and I led you for two seconds of meditation, you would go right back and say, "Wow, that was great." When my vibrating rhythm is affecting you, that's magnetism, because I've practiced so long. If one takes energy in the right way, to the right center, with the right values, it's very profound. I'm not looking for another religion to replace anyone's religion. I'm looking to put them in direct contact with the Boss, with the divine consciousness.

Do cave monks sitting and meditating serve a vital purpose?

It works for very few people. If you go to a cave and you cut yourself out of life, you can reach enlightenment, but you're not using life for your lessons. You have gone a very extreme way. It definitely works, but it's hard. It's almost painful.

How is it helping the planet to evolve? You singularly can't evolve. We're all a mass of energy. I can't evolve without the whole universe evolving with me. How can I help the whole universe evolve quicker? Get yoga to them, because their evolution is connected to mine. We are all connected behind the mind on a more subtle level. Every time I meditate, yes, I do evolve the planet. But every time the planet meditates, they're evolving me. Let's get the planet meditating.

By changing yourself, you change the world. But we mustn't forget the other concept. By changing the world, we change our Self,

too. It's the second part that's very important. Take your enlightenment back into life and spread it into life. Weave your divinity like
a thread in a tapestry. Weave your divinity into life.

Alan Finger, founder of Yoga Zone, began his path in yoga
over thirty-five years ago under the tutelage of his father,
Mani Finger. His father studied both at home in South Africa
and on regular travels to India, a study that transformed his
own life and that of his son. Since the age of fifteen, Alan has
dedicated his life to the in-depth study of various yoga traditions, leading to the development of *Ishta* yoga, a physical
and spiritual form of yoga, addressing the individual needs of
each who practices it. Alan resides in Westchester, New York
with his family.

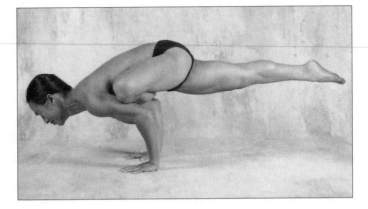

RODNEY YEE
O A K L A N D

What was your introduction to yoga?

The thread starts when my dad got me into gymnastics around nine or ten. I remember having a difficult time in gymnastics, because I had a very stiff body. I was already looking at other bodies and trying to figure out why some people could do what they could do and other people couldn't. I had an eye for looking at the physical body, and understanding form and restrictions from an early age. When I was about five or six, I had a friend next door. He could sit like a lot of kids can, where they are sitting with their thighs parallel and their calves perpendicular to their thighs. It looks like their legs are broken. I couldn't do that as a kid. I thought, "Why does his legs move like that and mine don't?"

I was very mechanically oriented. I would fix my mom's music boxes at age five. Up until the eighth or ninth grade, I wanted to become an engineer or a mathematician. In high school, I started switching things around. I became much more socially interested. Not just girls, but more interested in social interaction in society at large. I had a philosophical nature, so I was always wondering. During my teenage years, like anyone else, I was going through a time of strong alienation and isolation. Having a philosophical nature, I was reading a lot of existentialism. Hermann Hesse had an influence. I read *Siddhartha* and his whole litany of books. I was on the high school gymnastics team—still dealing with a very difficult body, but performing okay.

I went to the University of California, Davis, and started taking ballet class, because I thought it would make me more flexible. I fell in love with dance. I was a physical therapy major at U.C.-Davis. I had a couple of internships, one at Easter Seals in Sacramento and one at Fairmont Hospital in Oakland. I really wasn't that interested, because I was dealing with stroke patients. As a young kid full of energy, it seemed slow. I took a contemporary ethics class at U.C.-Davis and loved that. During the summertime, I had taken an apprenticeship at Oakland Ballet, and they had offered me a position with the company. So I transferred to U.C.-Berkeley's philosophy department and was a classical ballet dancer.

After a year, the company wanted me full-time, so I quit the philosophy department to pursue ballet. I knew dance was something I had to do when I was young, and I really was interested in pursuing it. I danced with the Oakland Ballet from 1977 to 1981. I started taking yoga in 1980, because I was still inflexible. Even though I was a ballet dancer, and I was stretching all the time and had some flexibility compared to people on the street, it was the very thing that was keeping me from pursuing dance further. A friend of mine and I took an Iyengar yoga class that was right upstairs from the ballet company. Since we were dancers, we could emulate the postures fairly quickly. Because of that, we got the benefits of yoga very quickly.

I remember after my first class being in disbelief at how good I felt on a mental, physical, and emotional level. I had a lot to compare it to, because I had been a dancer and a gymnast. It was hard to believe that I felt so good, because I had always done physical things. I had always studied philosophy. But I had never been able to merge my philosophy with actuality. I got a real intuition, even from my first class, that this made me feel at peace. It made me feel quiet. It made me feel incredibly healthy. It made me feel emotionally balanced.

I went to Japan to dance with the Matsuyama Ballet Company. Fortunately, another dancer in the company was also a yoga teacher. Like any dance company, during rehearsals you have a lot of time sitting around waiting for your part to come up. You're basically in the studio all day long rehearsing and taking class. During rehearsals, he would teach me yoga. It was a form called Oki yoga, which is named after a Japanese man, Oki, who went to India and studied yoga. He came out with a very vigorous form of yoga—long standing poses. Not that much different from Iyengar, really. He was a very dedicated and strong practitioner. Very orientated towards the *asanas* and *pranayama*. I stayed a year-and-a-half in Japan. I danced full-time, taught English, and studied yoga.

I came back to the United States in 1983 and studied yoga about three or four times a week. I was still dancing, but I didn't want to join a classical ballet company. There weren't many options in the Bay Area. There was either the Oakland Ballet or the San Francisco Ballet. I didn't have the body type for San Francisco. So it was a matter of joining my old company, getting out of dance completely, or doing modern and jazz locally. I decided to do modern and jazz. Because I didn't really need modern or jazz class and was working with local choreographers, I took yoga class. Suddenly, I was doing yoga every day, instead of dance class. I was practicing yoga with Donald Moyer three times a week and working out on my own. Working out was no problem, because I had developed a dance regiment. I was very diligent. Because I was familiar with philosophy, and familiar with working with my body in shapes and feeling things very intimately in my body, the yoga came very quickly. I soon began to realize it was a merging of everything I was interested in—the physical, the philosophical, and the emotional. Yoga took care of the whole package.

I asked Donald, after about two years of studying with him pretty rigorously, what the Iyengar Institute in San Francisco was like. I wasn't interested in becoming a teacher. I was just interested in studying more in depth than in public classes. He encouraged me to go there, and I went and found my next teacher, Manouso Manos. He really made my practice jump up another step. I went from five-minute headstands to twenty-minute headstands. I started realizing that my perception of the body was pretty keen after all these years. My perception of philosophy was developed. I started to realize that I was seeing other people's bodies as accurately as a lot of teachers. I thought, "This is what I want to do. This is what I want to teach. This is what I love."

It was the first thing in my life to which I had no emotional, intellectual, or physical resistance. In dance, there was always a philosophical resistance in that it was a lifestyle where people had no idea what they were doing. Sexual politics were crazy. There was no philosophy behind the practice of dance. It was dog eat dog in the performance world. There wasn't really a lifestyle. In gymnastics, there's not really a lifestyle. Physical therapy didn't have the philosophical or the spiritual aspects. It didn't seem to be addressing the emotional aspect of human beings. It was very scientific and tried to be void of emotion. It became very clear to me that yoga was something that really combined all of the things I was interested in.

Yoga was the first thing I studied that allowed me to more fully live the things I believed in. As a dancer, I philosophically believed in being a vegetarian. It was non-hoarding and being physically light. It was something I wanted to do, but I could never stick to a vegetarian diet when I was a dancer. When I started doing my *asana* practice, the postures started cleansing me to the point where I didn't desire meat. It wasn't something that I had to discipline myself to become. Becoming a vegetarian happened organically. Yoga brought me there without any discipline at all. It was the very first thing in my life that gave me hope I might achieve the ideals I thought were precious—non-violence, non-hoarding, non-stealing, honesty. I wanted to be honest after practicing. I just wanted to tell the truth. Yoga gave me the strength to do that. I was so taken by it. Yoga brought back hope. It brought the feeling I could realize my dreams.

When did you make the transition from yoga student to yoga teacher?

In 1985, after studying seriously for a couple of years, Donald Moyer asked me to teach a teenage class at the Yoga Room. Teaching came really easily. My family is good at communication. We're accurate at communication. We love people. My dad molded us to be in the service of other people, so service was a natural thing. Teaching was very natural. I was a waiter and a yoga teacher. I had been waiting tables when I was a dancer. I tell the teachers I am training that they should go be waiters and waitresses for a while, because it gets people to be quick. Your eye gets fast. It's a service-oriented job. I always make fun by saying that my days as a waiter really helped add up to being a yoga teacher.

What is your heritage?

I am Chinese. My father was born in China. My mother was born in the United States. They are both of Chinese descent. I am the youngest of five. I was born in California, spent my first nine years in Oklahoma, and three years in Puerto Rico. I've been in Oakland since I was twelve. Even though there was a lot of assimilation, we always ate Asian food. The feeling at home was very much one of our idea of Confucianism—respect the elders, etc. The feelings and teachings of the family that I grew up with were really quite Chinese. At the same time, we were very much American. It's a very interesting mix.

My dad was a pilot in the Air Force. He came to the states alone when he was twelve right in the heart of the Depression. He landed in El Paso, Texas. He was from a very small part of China called the Taishan area. The land was overfarmed. There was not a lot of ability to feed families. People were coming to the United States to send money back home to China. He learned English and Spanish, and went from kindergarten through high school in six years. He went to Texas A&M when he was eighteen and joined the reserves to pay for his college education.

I am sure you have deep respect for him.

Yeah, now that I am old enough to really look at him as a person. We had a very fiery relationship. When I became an adult, we could never be in the same household without screaming at each other. After doing yoga for about three years, I went home, and he began to go into his old spiel, "What are you doing with your life?" Blah, blah, blah. It was sort of insulting.

I was doing strange things for an immigrant family. I wasn't concerned about economics. I was into philosophy. I was in dance, then I was in yoga. It was very hard for a father who had worked so hard to support a family and had done a very good job of that. We were always butting heads. He was butting heads with all the other siblings who also were liberal-minded. Yoga got me to a place where I had no gut reactions to my father. Every time he was saying something against me, I had no gut-wrenching feeling where I had to get angry and stormy. I realized the man totally loved me. I could hear it. It wasn't in the words. It was underneath the words. I could relax to the point where I understood totally that he cared about me. Yoga produced such deep change in me, from that time on I could totally listen to my dad. Our relationship really changed. I was the first child out of five to have a decent relationship with him. I owe it all to yoga.

Julie Lawrence mentioned you practicing yoga with your kids climbing on you.

I now have a yoga room at home. We added on to the house. But before that there was a little strip of a hallway where I would do yoga with the kids on me. They still climb on me when I do my yoga, but now they're practicing themselves. I try to wake up a little earlier and get my main practice. There are aspects of yoga that are meant to be reclusive, but most of yoga is about relationship. Yoga means to bring together, to yoke. If it's going to bring things together, it's ultimately about relationship. It's about community. Yoga is deeply introspective, but it is also connecting with the world.

What do you hope to teach your children about yoga?

A big aspect of the practice is about respect. As a parent, my main responsibility is to teach my children to respect other people and respect the world at large—the environment, the animal kingdom, the plant kingdom. Respect is really a big thing a parent can teach a child. Other things will take care of themselves.

Watching me do yoga every day and then joining in, the kids have a much larger idea of what a person can be physically. It also gives them a sense of people being diligent about their work and loving their work. I hope to encourage my kids to do what they love.

Is that a different message than you heard from your father?

My father would tell us philosophically, "You do whatever you want in the world, as long as you can look in the mirror and be proud of yourself." And yet, on the other hand, he was very much a man for whom economics was an important part of life. He understood the role of economics. He would also be saying, "You've got to earn enough money to make a living and to take care of yourself." He saw a lot of people who didn't earn enough money and didn't take care of themselves during very hard times in this world. He knew what that could do to people. He was very concerned. But philosophically, money didn't concern him. It was confusing as a child, but I grew up respecting both things. It's good to make a living and it's good to follow your dreams.

Have you ever been the victim of racism?

Never in the yoga community, but I teach all over the world and get outside of the yoga circle. So, sure. The next racism that will be faced in this country will be the result of a cold war with China. There could be heavy racism against Asian people in years to come. A lot of threat will be coming from Asia now, instead of Russia. For black people in this country, there is incredible racism. Maybe insurmountable, unless we teach our children differently. Race will always be something that people will use as a dividing line. It's so undeniable. People have a hard time closing those gaps.

I would like to see the United States realize that it needs to fos-

ter a sense of cohesiveness, a sense of getting along, a sense of getting together, not a sense of isolation where people are individually
doing their own thing. One of the things we need is a community
to belong to. It's a big challenge. The only possible solution I see is
people having dinner with different races every day. Literally sitting
down, having dinner together, and getting to know each other. Not
through political mandate, but through people being with people.

*What wisdom can you share that you have garnered from the different
places you have traveled and lived?*

The wisdom comes from seeing that there are a lot of ways to
live life. There are a lot of ways to structure life, but I have seen a
lot of incredible similarities about being a human being. There are a
lot of similarities about what people consider respect.

I go to Bali every year. Bali is a place where people live in a
really incredible way. They live in small villages. They have a
strong community. They live close to the earth, but they also live as
artists, musicians, and dancers. Art and spirituality are extremely
woven into everyday life. That is one thing I would hope we could
do as Americans. Life is not about working and making the numbers bigger in the bank account. It's about living your own individual dreams.

We're a very challenged and troubled nation. We need to start
learning how to take care of ourselves. We should really figure out
what we need as human beings and what takes care of us holistically.
We're lacking cohesiveness as a nation. We are a mixture of many different cultures and many different moods. There is a lot of beauty in
that, but there are unbelievable challenges. I have seen many different
countries. I have been to Europe, Japan, and India where there is a lot
more homogeny in the culture. There is a lot of beauty that comes out
of that. There are a lot of things that people don't have to question.

Questioning is a great thing, but in the United States, we have made it a way of life. If you question everything and you have so many choices about everything, ultimately your mind gets inundated with choices and decisions. Even something as simple as what kind of food you are eating tonight. If you're in Bali, you eat Balinese most every day of your life. What video are you going to rent? What movie are you going to see? In most countries, there aren't that many questions. I come back to the United States and I hear all these mental challenges. We've got to decide *everything*. There are so many different things to consider. It creates confusion. It's a good thing to have choice, but it can actually be very debilitating.

Perhaps out of all this choice could come a choice of simplicity.

People are making that choice nowadays, but it's still cloaked. People want to simplify by moving to the country, but they end up moving their city life to the country, instead of really simplifying. A lot of people are not willing to give up. We have not been philosophically taught that giving things up is good. We come from an immigrant mentality, from not having much on the table. That's our ancestry. It doesn't matter whether you're Polish, German, English, French, Chinese, Mexican, or African. We all came here as immigrant families. Putting food on the table was really important. We came trying to figure out a new way. That's America's history. It has a very important ramification on our present way of thinking about our future. We have not been taught to say, "Less is more." We come from the mentality of "Gather for the winter. Have something in reserve." It's not this way in every culture in the world. There are cultures where one is taught not to hoard.

Do you think there is any correlation between hoarding and Americans being overweight?

It's the same exact psychology—excess. Do everything in excess, because pretty soon, you may be without. Most of us are running way too fast and way too much. We don't have very much contact with the earth or an element of grounding in our lives. We've never praised that. Ballet is a perfect example. Everything in classical ballet is up and airy. In Christian philosophy, everything that is cleaner and divine is up above the earth. Everything that is dirty and evil is of the earth. We have been taught, "Don't be of the earth."

Food grounds you. When people put on extra weight, they ground themselves. Important businessmen and businesswomen are overweight, because that's the only way that they can ground all of the activity that's running though them. If they were lithe and light, they wouldn't be doing half the stuff they are doing in the first place. The overweight problem in the United States is very much related to our history, our ideology, and our philosophy.

The preferred image in the United States is an overweight man who is very powerful. Not only in the United States, but in other cultures as well. In China, they bound women's feet. If you had your feet bound, that meant you were wealthy. If you were pale and overweight, you were not in the fields working. You didn't have to work as a peasant. It comes from being in a time when there wasn't excess. You wanted to save. Now we're destroying. Through our excess the opposite is happening. If we continue this excess, it's actually going to threaten our survival as the human race.

America represents five percent of the Earth's population, and we consume thirty-three percent of its natural resources. All the other countries are trying to catch up with us. I teach yoga to environmental scientists. All of them tell me that if China, with a billion people and one-fifth of the world's population, came up to the American standard of living, the world would be destroyed in less than five years. This is fact, not theory.

What are we proposing as a leading nation? We're saying, "You want to consume. Everyone must have their own car. Everyone has to have all of this." Well, the world can't do that. The world will not sustain that. A battery has a limited amount of energy. Earth is a little battery. It's a contained element. It can't run what we're asking it to do. Somewhere along the line, our survival actually depends on our ability to change this whole idea of hoarding. Our generation is confronted with the exact opposite problem that our ancestors had. And yet, it's the same problem—the problem of survival. The facts are undeniable. The facts are that we are overusing the environment, and the environment will have the last say.

Rodney Yee is the co-director, along with his wife, Donna Fone, of the Piedmont Yoga Studio founded in 1987. He was a ballet dancer with the Oakland Ballet Company and the Matsuyama Ballet Company of Tokyo. Rodney studied philosophy and physical therapy at the Universities of California at Davis and Berkeley. He has studied with yoga master B.K.S. Iyengar in India and is featured in the award-winning *Yoga Journal's* "The Yoga Practice Series" videos. He teaches workshops internationally and teacher training intensives nationally. Rodney resides in Oakland with his wife and his three young children.

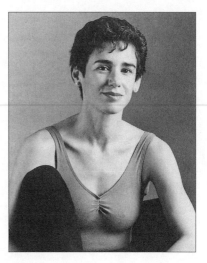

DONNA FARHI
CHRISTCHURCH, NEW ZEALAND

You're American, but you wouldn't guess that by your accent.

I have a chameleon-like accent. I was born to a non-practicing Jewish father, so my name is fifteenth century Spanish Hebrew, and a non-practicing Catholic mother in New Jersey. We moved many times, but I spent most of my early childhood in San Pedro, California. At the age of ten, my father decided we would be best off living in New Zealand, a country none of us had ever been to. We didn't even know anyone there. I lived in New Zealand from age ten to twenty and was very unhappy there. I returned to the United States, but now I find myself through a very strange *karmic* situation, once again living in New Zealand. I go back and forth between the two countries. I am in New Zealand eight months of the year, and I am teaching in other parts of the world, mostly the United States, but also in Mexico and Europe, for four months of the year.

Are your parents still living in New Zealand?

My mother and all my brothers and sisters live in New Zealand. My father has returned to the United States. They are very happy there, but it was a difficult country for me.

Why?

When we moved to New Zealand, it was one of many moves for our family within a period of seven years. My father had wanderlust and was always looking for a better situation. Within a few months of being there the family was thrust into a crisis. My mother became very ill, so at the age of ten, I was effectively left without parents. My mother was not well. My father was very much into his work. He has the IQ of a genius, but he doesn't know how to connect with people. I found myself in this strange culture that I did not fit into. There wasn't one person that I could speak to about what was going on with me.

At age ten, it would be difficult to verbalize your feelings.

Very difficult to verbalize, especially in a family atmosphere where the message was implicit that we were not to speak about my mother's illness. Her illness was crucial in my whole formative process, because very early on I had to develop an incredibly strong inner-reference system. I was introduced to yoga at high school in New Zealand when I was sixteen. At that time, it was a really weird thing to do. Only the very strange kids would sign up for something like yoga. Everyone else was off ice skating or doing something popular. I went to the class, and it was such a powerful experience for me. By the time I had walked home from school that day, I decided yoga was something I wanted to do every day.

In a few days, I collected books including Richard Hittleman's *Twenty-Eight Day Exercise Plan*. It doesn't tell you at the beginning that it's twenty-eight day increments for the rest of your life, but I bought his book and a few others. From that moment on I was practicing yoga every day by myself, which at the time didn't seem odd. But now that I am teaching, I realize it's extremely unusual for a girl of that age to be alone in a room for an hour-and-a-half a day practicing yoga.

As a teenager, did yoga provide a vehicle for you to look within?

I don't think it was as conscious as that. All I knew was that I felt good inside while I was practicing and so much of my experience outside of my yoga practice was one of fear. I was afraid a lot of the time when I was in New Zealand. My father was always coming up with these incredible plans for moving to New Guinea. Then it was Singapore. "Wouldn't be wonderful for the children to learn Chinese." I had this fear all the time that I was about to be picked up and moved somewhere else. The move to New Zealand had been so difficult. You couldn't have had two cultures more opposed in values than America and New Zealand.

Why?

In America, it's a crime to be a failure. In New Zealand, it was a crime to be a success. It's changed now, but in those days you were taught within the school system and within the society not to stand out. You were not to express yourself. You were not to do anything that showed your passion or excitement for life. And if you felt that, you should mute it in some way. You should turn the volume down on the inner-life excitement that you had. I had a tremendous amount of it. I was vivacious and had a ferocious appetite for learning. The teachers were discouraging me from learning.

During that period, I felt as if I was living on some other planet with people whose language I did not understand, and they did not understand my language. But yoga is a universal language. During practice I felt I was entering this universal language, and communicating with myself and with my larger Self at the same time.

Did you have the feeling that the moves were about your father and not really about the kids, but that was the spin on it?

Yes. It wasn't about us at all. My father was a person who never realized that he was taking himself wherever he went, and his unhappiness was intrinsic to his own being. It wasn't the job. It wasn't the country. It wasn't the people. He could have been dropped into paradise and he still would have found something that wasn't working there for him. We were the baggage that got towed along on this very bumpy ride from place to place.

Where is your father today?

He's very alone. He's still drifting.

And his forwarding address?

The last time I checked he was in Kentucky. That tells you something.

Did you think yoga would be your profession?

When I was sixteen, I was involved in theater and I thought that would be my profession. It became apparent as I worked with theater that movement would be the axis of my theater. As I looked for ways to develop that part of myself, I started studying dance in New Zealand. Within about a year-and-a-half, I decided I wanted to come back to the United States. I auditioned for the California Institute of the Arts dance program in Valencia and got a scholarship to study there.

After a year, I returned to San Francisco and studied dance in the studios there for many years. I was practicing yoga during that time, but it was in the background. I reached a point with dance where I felt I had become a perfect little machine that could do all of these clever things with my body, but I had no inner life anymore. I found it very difficult to exist in the dance community. I was a young woman suffering from anorexia, and it was not a very healthy community to belong to. When I was getting ready to look at dance companies, I started experiencing intense pseudo-cardiac symptoms. I say pseudo-cardiac symptoms, because none of the doctors could find anything wrong with my heart. But I would have searing pains where I couldn't breathe in or breathe out. I literally couldn't function anymore as a dancer. I didn't quite know what was going on in my psyche.

After doing all of these tests, one doctor said, "I think you're suffering from a broken heart." That made a lot of sense to me. I couldn't do this movement system which I loved with all my heart. I couldn't dance from my inner life in a healthy way. I couldn't find a place for myself in that world where dance could be the expression of my spirit, rather than simply a technical game. I walked home from the studio one day and I decided that I couldn't go on. I stopped cold turkey. It was a real crisis for me. I spent many months being really quiet and trying to feel. My heart symptoms started to abate, and I started to feel better.

Yoga had always been something solid for me. I needed to find my inner life again. So I decided I would study yoga. I chose the system of yoga that would perpetuate my obsession with perfection and form. I went to the Iyengar Yoga Institute and entered their teacher training program. At that time, their teaching program was very exciting. There was a very open atmosphere, and the faculty was fabulous. It took me about three years to complete the two-year program, because I traveled to Greece, India, and England to study with other teachers as well.

Are you still teaching in the Iyengar tradition?

No, not at all.

Why?

I did with my yoga exactly what I did with my dance. I repeated the same lesson. I took it to the nth degree, as far as form went. I was extremely aggressive in my practice. I wanted to be able to do all these really difficult things. It was the same kind of attitude that I brought to my dance, and I arrived at the same place—another crisis where I felt that my practice had become extremely mechanical.

At the same time, I had an intuition during my practice that there was another way to practice that would honor my inner life. Sharing that with others within the Iyengar system became very difficult. Towards the end of my training as a teacher, it was made clear that the organization was changing. The word *guruji* was springing up. The idea of having a guru and propagating this system of knowledge was in place. They were closing their doors to any outside influences. You weren't supposed to study with anybody who wasn't an Iyengar teacher. Suddenly there was this exclusion of outside information. To expand beyond the framework of what was defined as Iyengar yoga was forbidden. The price for that was that I would be put outside the village gates.

For a long time, I sat on the gate and swung back and forth. That's anyone's great fear—to be put outside the village gates. As a child, having been outside the village gates with a whole culture, I was tremendously fearful of following my heart. At a certain point, I decided that was the same question I had never answered with my dance. I had to be true to my heart. I broke away from the Iyengar system. For a while it was difficult. When you leave an organization, you see yourself in reference to it. As I began to find my own center of gravity, I no longer saw myself in reference to it. I am thankful for the information I was given. I use it as a structural platform for some of the things I do, but I don't adhere to the methodology in my teaching anymore.

The people who came before me were Angela Farmer and Victor Van Kooten. I went to Greece to work with Angela and Victor. I discovered that their way of working had too little structure for me, but Angela gave me the courage to follow my heart. They paid a big price, because they were the first to step outside the gates publicly. I feel really indebted to both of them, because without their work, a lot of us might not have the courage to move in this new wave. The new wave is here. That's what's happening across the United States. Teachers, who have studied very thoroughly, sometimes thoroughly in many different traditions, are contributing to the evolution of yoga with new ideas and new methodologies— even rewriting yoga philosophy.

You went to India and studied with Mr. Iyengar.

Yes, I did.

Since you had not left the village gates at this time, was it a positive experience?

Before I went to India, I went to another country and studied with a teacher who worked extremely aggressively with me. We were working about five or six hours a day, six days a week. By the end of my stay with this teacher, I felt psychologically shattered. I thought the teacher knew everything. If the teacher wanted you to do something, that's what you did. By the time I got to India, I was completely unawed by Iyengar. I found the experience quite mild. After doing the classes with him and his daughter, Geeta, I would practice in my room, because it didn't feel like I had done enough for the day. He pretty much left me alone. I think he must have sensed that I had reached a threshold point and that any more input would have been an overload. He really didn't interact with me very much in India.

What I learned in India was how I don't learn. I can honestly say that I do not remember any technique from the whole time I was there. Not any piece of information, other than I don't learn in an atmosphere of fear. That lesson has really affected my own teaching, because I always begin with creating a safe, sacred place. When people feel safe, they can make enormous changes. They will go very deep with you, because you have established trust. Safe means the student has the right not to do something. The student can stop when they feel they have had enough. They won't have their personal boundary transgressed in any way. There are all kinds of parameters for safety, but people know when they feel safe. That is the precursor to working with anyone in the group—everyone feels very safe.

When you work with people on a very organic level, and you provide a situation in which they can explore the inner connections in their body and explore the relationship between parts of the body, people find an alignment that is functional and healthy for them in that moment. Rather than having a picture of a posture in their mind or even emulating what I'm demonstrating at the front of the room, they are trying to find how they can inhabit that posture in a healthy way. Everyone has different body proportions and different difficulties with their body, different mobilities and immobilities. At any given moment, the form is going to look different for each individual, even breath to breath. The form is going to be changing.

The idea of one correct way of doing *asana* is unsound. When the form is more important than the person practicing the form, then you've lost the plot. That's not the goal anyway. The goal is for each and every individual to find their Self. If you can use the form as a means to doing that—fine. But once a person thinks that the form is the goal, that's the big mistake. That's not the goal.

The truth of yoga, when I can live it, is that the state of unification exists now. It is not a state that I have to strive towards. That state is already functioning within me. My work is to see the ways in which I am not realizing it. I ask my students, "Will you let yourself be moved?" The question changes from "Why can't I do this movement?" to "What am I doing to stop myself from being moved by life?"

How we exist in ourselves during practice is how we're going to function when we're off the mat. Let's say I'm in the habit of always holding my shoulders together, so that when I breathe, my shoulders can't move, my arms never move, and my chest never expands to the side. It's not that I need to learn how to breathe into my chest. I would breathe into my chest, if I would undo all the things that I'm doing to stop that movement from happening. I would be in a state of co-participation with my breath.

Where do the things that inhibit movement come from?

It's an interesting question. The most fascinating questions that I'm playing with right now are, "Why do people hold their breath?

Why do they stop their spine from undulating when they breathe? Why do they stop all these organic movements that are happening when a person is relaxed? Why do they stop these things from happening when they're in postures?" The answer that I've been coming up with is that the desire for certainty is so great, we will bend reality towards having certainty versus being dynamically alive.

"Do you want to be dynamically alive?" That's the choice I present to students. It means you throw yourself in there, and you are moved around. It's going to be wonderful, because you are feeling vital when you are dynamically alive. Or, "Do you want certainty?" Yes, you will find answers. You will find perfectly correct ways of doing your postures and your practice. You will find structures. And you will barricade yourself from life. Life isn't this tidy little package where you know where everything goes. Life is intrinsically changing and dynamic.

What does the desire for control stem from?

Fear. Where does tension come from? Tension comes in my body when there is some challenge asking me to change. If I don't want to change, there is going to be tension. The paradox, for most of us, is that while the situation we are in isn't terribly great, we are holding onto it because we think the one to come is going to be even worse! Nine times out of ten, it's far better than anything we could imagine. In *asana*, when people let go of their very strong ideas about the way everything is, they find that the expression of that *asana* is so much more profound than anything they could have imagined with their logical mind. Once people have a taste of that, it's very hard for them to go back to searching for authoritative answers or correct positions. It's very hard for them to go back to practicing in a mechanistic way, because the other is so pleasurable. Pleasure should be the motivation in a practice, not pain, not punitive discipline, not doing it because we ought to. It's right for us, because it's pleasurable.

I found *pranayama* extremely frustrating and unpleasant. That doesn't necessarily have to be a part of *pranayama* as a practice, but the way it was taught to me was mind over matter. It wasn't until I did a *Vipassana* workshop in San Francisco, where we were asked to simply let our breath do whatever it was going to do, let whatever thoughts we had arise and dissolve without manipulation, that I realized how difficult that was for me. The *Vipassana* meditation was revolutionary. I stopped practicing *pranayama*. I say I don't do *pranayama*, but I think I do another form of it. I'm practicing a neo-classical revival of the initial intention of yogis, which was to enter the *pranic* life force, rather than be separate from it.

Control is easy for me. I was a control freak, and yoga is a perfect practice for a control freak. What was difficult was to stop manipulating. The question came up, "Why am I manipulating and controlling myself in this way?" What came out of that question was that there was a whole underworld within myself, a whole dark shadow that I wasn't living in, that I was denying and suppressing all the time while I was practicing yoga. As positive as my yoga practice had been in many ways, it had also been used as a means to suppress this shadow.

I became captivated by the question of what is natural breathing. What is the essential nature of breathing? That question is still with me today. I'm still exploring it. I'm exploring what is natural movement. How does a human body move naturally? Those questions involved a complete restructuring of my psyche, because I had to look at all the material I had been suppressing. That was another really difficult time for me.

What material were you suppressing?

I realized that my need to have everything under control came from a childhood where I felt completely out of control. My need to manipulate situations and my practice, so that everything was structured and predictable, had to do with very deep fears of unworthiness and a fear of self-annihilation. If I let go even for a second of this structure holding me up, I would be annihilated.

Your suppression may have been a very valuable defense mechanism growing up, but it appears you outlived its usefulness. It became a limitation.

Exactly. Quite often when students come into an intensive with me, their first reaction will be one of refusal. I always watch the ones who have the hardest time in the first day with the organic work that we're doing. Usually by the second or third day, they're having an emotional crisis. They are having that crisis because the investment to hold onto what they know is so great. There is fear underneath. If they are courageous enough and they feel safe enough, they are going to meet that material head on. By looking at it, by embracing the fear, the anger, the pain, whatever it is, they are going to be a lot more alive than they were through suppressing it.

When you stop manipulating and imposing ideas about how a form should be, and start listening to what the body is saying, you will open yourself to the information of these natural movement patterns. That information is so much more powerful and logical than anything you could think up with your linear mind, if you are willing to be a vehicle for that expression. The movement takes on a life of its own, and the person doing the movement is no longer there. There's no disassociation.

Yoga in this country is practiced as disassociation, of mind telling body what to do, of mind telling breath what to do. We have done that with nature and we have seen the results. We thought we were so clever that we knew when to move a dam or when to spray a field with pesticides. But when you stop long enough to really listen to the ecology of the body and the environment of the body, you hear a phenomenally complex, beautiful, whole, balanced organism. Tapping into that is the practice.

Is the beginning of this organic work the awareness of the breath?

It's the precursor. You have to have self-perception. There has to be cultivation of some kind of self-reflective consciousness. Without that, you can't really begin the work.

What wisdom and understanding have you learned through your breath work?

I don't think of it as breath work, which is strange for somebody who's written a book called *The Breathing Book*, but you have to call it something! Breathing is movement. I teach movement.

What have I learned? It's not a matter of overcoming fear; it's living with it. Practicing yoga doesn't mean you answer your questions. It means you learn to live with your questions, rather than having some kind of righteousness that you've answered them. You remain open-minded all the time, because there may be another possibility that you haven't considered.

You have obviously remained open-minded by returning to New Zealand.

If you asked me five years ago if I would ever live in New Zealand again, I would have said, "Never. It's the last place on the face of the earth I will ever put myself again." I went back to the place where all the demons were—and that was truly healing. *Karmically*, for me to go back to New Zealand was perfect, because I went back to the place where my fears began. They weren't really that developed before I left the United States as a ten-year-old. I did a lot of family archeology. I had a lot of talks with my mother and my family, and we're cultivating a new family since my going back to New Zealand. I'm actively seeking out relatives I've never met. I went to New York to meet my cousin. I brought my aunt back to New Zealand last year. She had not seen my mother in thirty years. I'm creating another family—the family that I want to have.

I feel grateful there have been people throughout the centuries who have passed on the practice of yoga. I am grateful for my family, and I think my family is grateful I am practicing yoga, because without the awareness I learned through the practice, I don't think the changes that have taken place in our family structure could have happened.

Donna Farhi is a Registered Movement Therapist who has been practicing yoga since she was sixteen years old. Her work has been informed and inspired by such great teachers as Judith Lasater, Dona Holleman, Angela Farmer, and most recently the work of Bonnie Bainbridge-Cohen. She leads workshops and teacher trainings throughout the world. Donna is a writer and columnist for *Yoga Journal*, and is the author of *The Breathing Book*. She is the co-director The Hatha Yoga School of Sumner in Christchurch, New Zealand with her partner Mark Bouckoms.

Donna loves to cook and dabble in the soil of her cottage garden. Her primary teacher for the last three years has been her thoroughbred gelding, Braga.

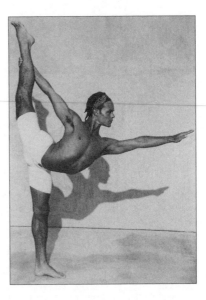

BARON BAPTISTE

BOSTON

Please describe your yoga heritage.

Nearly sixty years ago my father, Walt Baptiste, founded San Francisco's first yoga center. His father introduced him to yoga. Some of these great early yoga teachers would come over here and connect with my dad. They stayed at our home when they came to San Francisco.

My forefathers were spiritualists looking for enlightenment and greater meaning in life. They were very much on the Eastern path. My grandfather connected with Vivekananda when Vivekananda first came to America. My grandfather's father was interested in early Eastern mysticism. My cousin, Charya Bernard, connected with Paramahansa Yogananda and was very close to him. My cousin was one of Yogananda's *Brahmacharyas*, or public representatives, and a real dynamic guy. I never met Yogananda. He passed away before I was born, but my father knew Yogananda pretty closely.

My roots are in *raja* yoga, or the "royal path," which is a lifestyle of seeking spiritual fulfillment, not just hatha yoga, even though my thrust now is teaching hatha yoga and yoga exercise for physical health and well-being. I use the yoga poses as a vehicle to teach the higher principles of *raja* yoga, and to cleanse and purify the mind and body to prepare a person for meditation and self-awareness.

When did you first visit India?

At a young age, my parents took me to India and I spent quite a bit of time there. When I was twelve, my parents left me there for a few months. I lived in Swami Rama's *ashram* in Rishikesh for about a month and then I went over to Kurpal Singh's *ashram* during the Kumbha Mela in Hardiwar.

The Kumbha Mela takes place every twelve years in India. It's the biggest spiritual event in the world. People come from thousands of miles all over India and countries outside of India. Several million people all come to this one place on the Ganges River. In *The Autobiography of a Yogi*, Yogananda talks about the Kumbha Mela and the cave yogis who kneel and kiss the ground every step. Some of them have done it for thousands of miles. They stop and kiss the ground every step.

Maybe that's why the Kumbha Mela is once every twelve years. It takes them six years to get back and start over.

Exactly.

What are your memories of visiting India as an adolescent?

It was a wonderful experience. I lived in an *ashram* for boys when I was twelve years old. Two or three hundred young boys all between the ages of nine and fourteen lived there. The boys that I stayed with were from the heart. They were beautiful. All had shaved heads and wore robes, and they were being trained to be *Vedantic* monks.

That experience changed my life. Even though my parents led a different lifestyle and had a different philosophy, to come out of America and live in that culture and environment gave me discipline. American kids are spoiled, and they can be mean-spirited and very competitive. There's very much of a one-upmanship at whatever age. "I've got toys that you don't have." It starts early and I don't know if it ends.

All the way to who has the biggest tombstone.

How much did Howard Hughes take to the grave with him?

I heard a Southern gentleman put it this way: "I've never seen a hearse pulling a U-haul."

Exactly.

Also, when you're a child you see through a lot of things. I would see seekers congregating at certain *ashrams* and to certain teachers almost under a hypnotic trance. The people got caught up in the guru and lost themselves, rather than finding their own Self. In fact, they were escaping from looking at themselves. I believe real gurus lead you to your inner Self.

Growing up in and around yoga from a young age has given me two perspectives. There's no question that I've derived some life-giving, life-sustaining, and life-saving principles and techniques and understanding about life. But there can be so much hypocrisy. I can also see through the dark side of yoga and realize that not everybody spouting truths and so-called paths to self-enlightenment is really who they are claiming to be. I have definitely seen the shadow side, as well as the light.

It's like the difference between Christianity and Churchianity. Human beings tend to get their hands on things and defile them and twist them, and keep continually justifying why they are changing them to fit their needs. Their needs may be based on total denial of their own personal issues, so they make everything fit them, rather than fitting the essence of what yoga is all about.

It's very common for people who were raised in a well-defined spiritual tradition to rebel. Did you experience a season of rebellion?

Absolutely. When I entered my teens, I started connecting with the world. I was into martial arts, surfing, and skateboarding. Peer pressure started to set in. Coming from such a unique background and family, there was a part of me that felt empty and different. It made me want to fit in. That's what most teens are grappling with, not to be themselves, but to fit in with a group.

My dad was a guru. He had a lot of followers and devotees. He had a large health and yoga complex. I had healthy influences, but I wasn't on some path to seek enlightenment. Just because I was born into that environment, it doesn't mean I was there by choice. Some people say you choose your parents. I don't believe that. I think there is *karma*, and maybe we are put into a specific situation for a purpose or reason. I don't know if we choose that as much as it's determined for us. My situation was not necessarily fulfilling for a young boy. I was trying to find my own identity in the world.

I had pain because my parents were busy. They were traveling a lot. A part of me felt an emptiness from not really truly connecting father-to-son versus guru-to-disciple. I wasn't looking to be a disciple—I just wanted my dad. He's a beautiful man. I suppose that left me more vulnerable to a lot of outside forces in the world that came from other friends who felt the same emptiness with their families and their homes. We would come together to create our own family, but being young egos, we were filtering in all the dark things like pot, drinking, and cigarettes.

Having and knowing higher spiritual principles created more conflict and anxiety for me. You have a conscience. The word con-science is "con" meaning "with," and "science" which is "to know." "With knowing." You know better. Your conflict is even greater because you know it's not the right path. Even though you're in conflict, you're doing negative things because you have pain. That pushed me even further over the edge. Then you become caught up in the cycle of trying to numb pain and creating more pain that you need to escape from. Usually when you're a teenager, meditation isn't an option. That's when you need a dad who will sit there and talk with you—that's the meditation for a teenager or a little boy.

What brought you home?

Going out into the world on my own and suffering. I had enough pain that I finally said, "I know about higher principles. What am I rebelling against, and what is the emptiness that keeps me rebelling?" Higher principles were ingrained into my nervous system and psyche from being raised with them from such a young age. The realization came that I just had to slam on the brakes and face the music. I believe that every person needs to find the truth on their own. Even though I was raised in a spiritual tradition, I needed to find it for myself. Hearing the truth intellectually is not enough. It's just words, verses and chapters, information and knowl-edge. It's got to trickle down from the head into the heart and become something you really live and not just talk about.

Living the truth is really what changes you. Then it becomes yoga. It becomes a path versus studying it, having it in your head, and being able to parrot it. If you have children, you bring a light to those children that introduces them to their light and allows them to live their life. You are helping bring more light to the world. That's yoga. It's not about how well you bend, or how many legs you can get behind your head, or how many *asanas* you have perfected and refined. It's much more about what you bring. Are you being a representative of the light?

I had a second rebellion. At twenty years old, I really got into my yoga practice. Every day I was doing three hours of intense hatha yoga. I began fasting and internal purification. I was meditating two hours every morning. Going to yoga classes all the time becomes a numbing of pain. You're just looking to feel good in yoga class and forget all your problems, but you start to realize that doesn't take care of the problems in your life.

I was really living for myself. *Totally.* My yoga practice was all about feeling. I was creating highs. It wasn't about other people or the world or anything other than me feeling good and finding peace away from the world, not peace with the world. I was not finding peace in daily situations, calm in the midst of chaos, or grace under pressure. It was an escape. I was very self-centered. It was the equivalent of going up into the Himalayas and living in a cave, but within the context of an American lifestyle.

Gandhi said, "If I could persuade myself that I could find God in a Himalayan cave I would proceed there immediately." I agree with Gandhi. There's no doubt in my mind that God lies and truth lies within humanity. We live in a world of conflict, and we are constantly dealing with stresses and pressures. Those things are lessons because they give us an opportunity to respond properly, not react, and the ability to see problems as mirrors of ourselves.

Did you want to teach yoga?

I did not want to teach initially. When I was a teenager I taught kids' classes. When I was eighteen, my dad pushed me into teaching a meditation class. I didn't really want to, but it was his class, and he was going away. I got resentful and angry, but after I actually taught the class and saw what he pushed me into, a thankfulness came over me. I realized that his pushing me to teach was good for me. He would always say, "You have a lot of important information. You should be willing to share it, not be so closed up." A part of me always thought that. I just didn't want to own it. But teaching that class was a beautiful experience.

What principles and techniques have you learned that you would not have learned or discovered without yoga?

That's an incredible question and important question to me, because I have looked at that, being around it for most of my life. Not long ago, I took a trip to my father's retreat center in Central America on the beach in El Salvador. It's beautiful. I love going down there with the family once a year. The last time I was down there it was quiet. There was no one around. The beach was empty, and it was a time where I could just be with myself. And the thought came to me, out of everything I have learned and done and seen, what is the one anchor I have taken that allows me to live yoga? To walk a path where I am actually unfolding as a human being, not just caught up in patterns and habits, and in my compulsions and blind spots? What is it that allows me to be in a process where I am, at whatever speed, unfolding and opening up as a person? Ultimately, for me, the most important thing is the ability to sit still on a daily basis. Sit still and wrestle with my inner person and gain some distance from that worldly, sensual creature that resides within me—to gain a little distance from ego.

It's the thinker watching the thinking, and going even beyond the thinker into the realm of stillness where I am watching the thinker, which is a part of me. This onslaught of mental chatter and unending conversation that takes place in the mind isn't me. The majority of people have the same types of thoughts, which take different forms, shapes, and flavors because of the individual's experiences. Usually self-doubt is a major factor within the thinking process. I have found that the ability to separate from ego has given me the ability to recognize the lie.

I have been able to see all these little denial mechanisms that distract me from the stillness. As I have been able to see it in myself, I also have been able to recognize it in other people. Not from a judgmental standpoint, but just recognizing things as they are. People are always reaching out. We are looking to cut the edge and to feel good. Trying to make ourselves feel good from the outside. By sitting still, even for a few minutes each day, the spiritual eye opens. I am able to see this ego nature and observe how it's being reinforced. The majority of people are seeking without even knowing that they are seeking, but they are looking for happiness in whatever ways they can justify it.

Why do people look outside themselves for happiness, instead of within?

It's a lack of understanding. You can even look at the word understanding—to stand under, to stand under something higher. There's a higher knowing, a higher guidance. When you are still and you are grounded in the moment, the present, you have this higher presence, which brings intuition and conscience.

If you look at this life from the beginning, we are born into turmoil and chaos. It's a painful world. Wherever the pain comes, there is pain that people have, just by the very nature of the human condition. Because we feel bad, we're looking to feel good, but we're looking in the wrong places. One way we try to fill emptiness is with food. That's why America has such a weight problem. We're smoking ourselves to death. Cancer. Heart disease. Most are diseases of lifestyle. We are looking outside for fulfillment, trying to collect more and more things, stuffing ourselves with more and more food. But it's all temporary fulfillment. We are left with a greater emptiness. We have more anxiety, and we reach even further to other things.

Does meditation alleviate the need for outside fulfillment?

Absolutely. When you sit, even if just for twenty minutes, you become fully aware of the rhythm of your breath and the waves of emotions traveling through the corridors of your body. You are heightening your awareness of those sensations. By being aware, you are separating from them. When you are not aware, you have gone into forgetfulness. Remembering is awakening. One of Buddha's disciples asked him, "Are you God?" Buddha said, "I am not God." The disciple said, "Are you a saint?" Buddha said, "I am not a saint." The disciple said, "Then what are you?" Buddha said, "I am awake."

To be still and to be present is faith. To know that in stillness higher knowing comes through. Contemplation comes after meditation. I am in a calmer zone, and I can contemplate my day. I can contemplate my relationship with my wife and my relationship with my boys. I see how I was impatient with my son when he wanted my attention. He wanted me. It allows me to deal with things nonjudgmentally, calmly, and patiently. I grow a little bit in each small situation that I deal with properly. I am creating a new pattern in my life and in the lives of other people.

When I am not handling things properly, I sit down. I sit with it and own it—not run from it. When I feel the churning and watch this separate energy moving through me, I realize it's not really me. It's in me, but it's not really me. By meditating, it's diffused. It's not being energized. I'm not throwing fat on the fire. Sometimes, the first fifteen minutes of meditation is pure pain. Then suddenly a warmth, a light, a peace comes over me. I am left in a different dimension, and I can walk through my life with more compassion and more understanding.

Just having a little distance, you start to see yourself. You see the sum total of all the experiences that made you as a person. These experiences don't own you anymore. You're not acting them out compulsively or subconsciously. You're not functioning from the unconscious; you're functioning from the conscious. Being in the moment, you start to recognize the truth, because you're standing in a different place within yourself.

Meditation brings me back to my center. It is my anchor. It's like the eye of the storm. Everything outside of us, even on the inside of us, is constantly churning and moving. Everything is fluctuating and changing. Within that there is stillness—a safe place— probably our only true stability in life.

How has becoming a householder affected your personal practice?

Getting married and then having kids was a big monkey wrench in my practice. That's what I thought initially. I realized the only reason it was a wrench in my practice was because my practice was all about me. Me, me, me. I resented it. I was angry. I went through that stage, then I realized, I am blessed because I have the opportunity to overcome my selfishness.

When my first child was born there were really two births—the birth of my child and the birth of me as a father. Discovering what that means has been profound. The most basic meaning is whatever limitations I have will be my sons'. My selfishness hurts me, but it hurts them as well. None of us can grow and have the opportunity to be who we can. I don't want to rob my sons of their birthrights.

My tendency is to relate to my boys in the same way I had a relationship with my father. In the first year of my oldest son's life, I was away a lot. I was walking in the footsteps of my father, even though I knew I wanted a different relationship with my son. Fatherhood has been a great challenge, because it is challenging the very core of my identity. It requires me to come out of my conditioning.

My children are mirrors of me. I can recognize myself as a young boy in them, and it does awaken the pain I had relating to my dad. It's easier for me to go out and seek success in the world, but it's a temporary fulfillment. The greatest fulfillment is slowing down and allowing myself to feel the pain of my childhood, and fulfilling my children in the way I truly wanted to be fulfilled.

Yoga has become more and more narrowed down to living life with myself and the inclination of my soul. Resolving it in myself begins with my family. If I can't deal with my own family properly—patiently and with understanding and connection—there is no way I can go out into the world and connect with other people.

Baron Baptiste was born into a lineage of yoga teachers. His father, Walt Baptiste, a former Mr. America, opened the first yoga center in California in 1935. Between the ages of twelve and twenty-two, Baron spent time living in various *ashrams* in the Himalayas where he undertook rigorous yoga training. He has developed an athletic style of fitness yoga based on the *Ashtanga*, Iyengar, and Bikram styles. He is seen by millions of Americans every day on his ESPN 2's "Cyberfit" fitness segments. Baron also hosts a popular Sunday morning radio show called "Your Personal Best." He teaches yoga internationally and at his Power Yoga Institute in Cambridge, Massachusetts, where he lives with his wife and two sons.

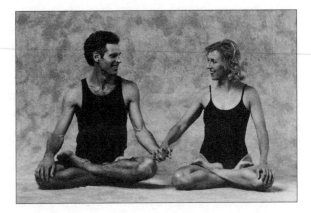

THOM AND BERYL
BENDER BIRCH

Thom, your first career was as a distance runner. How were you able to run great distances?

TB: Through meditation. Within my running career the one element that allowed me to focus and concentrate and really deal with being a competitor was meditation. The mind is the thing that's the hardest in running. Running is mostly mind. To do the physical training, you first have to do your mental training. To run twenty miles, you have to find peace, calm, and focus. Right before races I used to sit for two hours in a dark room with five specific colored candles and meditate.

      It's wonderful being a competitor, but the nature of being

in competition is not an easy thing. It really bombards the nervous system. It's not always best for the person, especially if you're a professional athlete or on a scholarship at a major university. When I was running for the University of Houston, the pressure was intense. Throughout my running career, I did meditation. I read Jean Couch's *Yoga for Runners*, and I had been doing transcendental meditation since the eighth grade, so by the time I got to college I already had a serious meditation practice.

When I got into *ashtanga*, it replicated my running because of the physicality. Heat is a constant companion of a distance runner, and being a New Yorker running in Houston, Texas, my first year was not spent competing against people, but competing against the heat. As a runner I always knew the *tapas* of heat was part of being healthy. Go for a ten-mile run. You feel clean, and you are clean. It's the same after an hour-and-a-half of *ashtanga*. You're clean. Your high is there.

What Beryl was teaching in yoga classes were things that I had to discover and learn to become a successful distance runner. That's really what drew me to her. If you look at the pictures of Krishnamacharya, B.K.S. Iyengar, and K. Pattabhi Jois as young men, they look like distance runners. We have a picture of Pattabhi Jois. He was long and lean and thin as a rail. If you read B.K.S. Iyengar's first autobiography, his time is filled with walking long distances. When I read about the yogis, I felt very akin. When I became a distance runner, it was the book *Siddhartha* by Hermann Hesse that made the most sense to me. I learned I would have to sacrifice to be a great runner. I would have to learn to eat little, to focus, to concentrate, and to be discriminate in terms of my energy. Running a hundred miles a week is being totally mindful because every ounce of energy matters.

Meditation allowed you to run a hundred miles a week. What was your motivation?

TB: To escape from my life. It was a way to get through college and out of New York City. My parents came from a very rough neighborhood. I grew up on the fringe, but my father and mother constantly brought me back to where they were born. My whole childhood was a rough, inner-city Bronx experience.

Beryl, was there a connection when you met Thom?

BBB: Yeah! The first time I saw Thom was in Houston, and I immediately started asking about him. We both noticed each other. His friend told me he was involved in a relationship, so I tried to put him out of my mind. Then we happened to see each other six months later in San Francisco. It seemed synchronistic. Here we were again, and this time Thom was just getting out of this other relationship. At that time, I had a prior obligation to go back to Colorado for about two weeks; otherwise, I probably would have stayed in San Francisco with Thom. It was fairly clear at that point that we were going to see each other again.

TB: We were both at a running conference in San Francisco. She was speaking about yoga for runners, and I was a race director. I was in dire straits. I ripped my Achilles tendon, and my doctor told me not to run and I would never run again. It had been over a year, and I was not recovering. I had a limp and my foot was immobile. I had just left a relationship, and I was despondent, thinking my life was over because my running was over. I was an athlete. I had a college degree, and I owned a running store, but my whole heart and soul since fourth grade had focused on being a professional athlete. I was at my peak. It was unbelievable how quickly it was over.

Being fit doesn't mean you're healthy. Being a great athlete doesn't mean you're healthy. Performance doesn't equal health. That was a hard thing to accept.

I took a couple of yoga classes with Beryl. She put her hand on my back, did something, and all of a sudden my whole body moved, and the tendon moved in a way that my doctor thought it never would. Having done yoga for fifteen years I see it was a miracle, and also a norm of things we see in yoga daily. The whole continuity of what *ashtanga* is really does set up a perfect situation to heal.

Beryl headed off to Colorado, and I went to Yosemite and stayed in a tent for three weeks training. I was running a hundred miles a week and trying to get my career back. Then I won a major 10K in San Francisco called the St. Jude's Race. St. Jude is a patron saint of hopelessness. I beat the defending champion by an inch. The next day, I was lame and not feeling well. I was supposed to go back to Texas, but I got on a plane to Colorado and went up to where Beryl was living in Fraser and found her. Beryl healed me. Three days later I asked her to marry me.

At the end of that summer, I ran in the national championships, finished in the top twenty, and was back on track. I regained my world class ranking. That blew my doctor's mind. I had another five successful years in my career and retired after winning a national championship.

That injury changed my life and was a true blessing. I was twenty-eight at the time. I had been running at a national level since age fourteen. I had maintained an international level for years. I meet Beryl fifteen months after surgery. I had been miserable for more than a year from having my career ripped out from underneath me. The injury saved my life and brought me out of a dark space into the light.

How is it being married to your teacher?

TB: It's very easy for me. I fell in love with her before she became my teacher. I have been trained since the fourth grade as an athlete. I was in training camps all summer. I competed all year. Beryl is one of the most knowledgeable teachers I have ever met, and I have been coached by some of the greatest coaches and been exposed to the greatest of the greats in the world of track and field.

Beryl, what led you to yoga?

BBB: From the time I was three years old, I recognized that things didn't happen by coincidence. I knew that I was here to evolve consciously. I remember formulating the idea that if, through my concentration, I could have a child born without a pinkie finger, that would be feedback that I had consciously evolved. I knew my evolution was my goal and my reason for being on this earth. I knew my reason for being was to express my divine nature.

I was born in October. As a child, I used to fantasize that I was the goddess of October. I was very much into ritual and pagan expressions of the goddess. I would wear capes and autumn leaves in my hair, and have diaphanous pieces of material hanging over my head or draped around my shoulders.

My mother died when I was fifteen. My father's influence came in for awhile. He was a Rhodes scholar with a Ph.D. in chemistry, so I thought I would be a chemist. When I got to college, because of severe unrecognized dyslexia, I could not comprehend physics, chemistry, or math. I managed to get A's in philosophy, religion, and literature. I had four emotionally catastrophic years at Syracuse University. I was frustrated and depressed. I was a cheerleader, and I have some happy memories, but I still have nightmares about unfinished business from college.

I got turned on to *ashtanga* yoga in 1963 when I took a course in Hinduism and *raja* yoga. It seemed like an ideal path. Then I didn't think about it again. It was a very difficult time, because I was struggling with being atheist on one side and having this very early spiritual experience as a child on the other. Yoga didn't come back to me until 1971 when I began studying with the Jains. Many Jains are practicing *ashtanga* yogis and follow the yogic path. They are also very governed by the principle of non-violence. For ten years I was very influenced by the practice of non-violence, and I read a lot of Mahatma Gandhi's teachings.

I went to India in 1974. I did not go to study with Pattabhi Jois. I went to study with some Jain monks and nuns. I did months of silence and *mendicant* walking from village to village. I traveled all over the north of India. I spent a month in Manali and a month in the Himalayas.

Thom, have you traveled to India?

TB: No. I think it would be a wonderful thing to do, but I feel absorbed in what's going on in the American yoga movement. In Cambridge, Massachusetts, we were doing a workshop, and an Indian man from Bombay spoke. He said only ten percent of the Indian culture is interested in yoga. The young Indians that I have met, some of the sons and daughters of gurus, convinced me that the wealth of yoga is in America. That's what I have come to feel and think with no disrespect to India, for without India, there would be no yoga.

BBB: They don't do yoga in India for health and fitness. It is a path of spiritual seeking. It's a method of self-realization.

TB: I feel I'm on the yogic path, but if I'm going to go to India, I want to come more to the end of my journey and be more evolved in my yoga practice.

BBB: I would like to go to some of the holy places with Thom. When I visualize us going, I don't visualize us going to study *asana*. I see us traveling. Going to Nepal and Bhutan. I would love to go to Ladakh and see some of the old Tibetan monasteries. Getting up, doing yoga, visiting some local person, and seeing the culture and history of this thing we do. Go as pilgrims really.

Some of the most memorable times I had in India were when I sat in the presence of the local guru who was either observing silence or fasting. These are people that are really trying to get it. They have observed silence for ten years. There's an anthill growing up around them. They are lying in a ditch for six years meditating on God. That kind of ascetic behavior doesn't go unrewarded. I think these people actually have vision. Maybe they can't materialize bananas, and maybe they can't bring the dead back to life, but they definitely have wisdom.

Those are the people who I would like to go and experience, even non-verbally. Just sit in their presence. I have had experiences in India that were very real. I lived in a little hut in Manali, where I understand there is now a Holiday Inn. There aren't many huts left and there aren't many remote corners of the world left. I would like to hit a few before this lifetime is over.

Speaking of before this lifetime is over, you had a wolf that saved your life.

BBB: That was Timber. If it hadn't been for Timber, I would have been frozen in a snowbank in Flagler, Colorado. My father had just died, and Timber and I were driving from New York to Colorado. It started snowing heavier and heavier and all of a sudden it was a full-out blizzard—a complete whiteout. I tend to be very prodigious and because of my dyslexia, I get very nauseous and sick to my stomach when I can't focus on the road in a whiteout. I can't drive in those conditions, because I start getting dizzier and dizzier, and sicker and sicker. I was driving and thinking, "Oh God, I can't do this. I've got to stop. I'll just pull over to the side of the road." We had a down sleeping bag and I thought, "I'll sleep and wait." Just as I was ready to stop, Timber jumped in the front seat, panting, and put his nose under my elbow. He was real agitated, and somehow I understood that he wanted me to keep going.

Five miles down the road there was this yellow light that was flashing in the little town of Flagler. A little "Motel, Motel" flashing light came up out of the snow. When we stopped, the wind was blowing eighty or ninety miles-an-hour. I couldn't get the door of the car open. Finally, I got it open, and Timber and I burst into this little log motel coffee shop. There was one room left, and we got it. They closed the road for three days. The morning of the third day, they opened the road and found people dead, frozen in their cars. You would drive down the road and look over and see a whole herd of cattle standing dead, frozen against the wind.

How is the practice of ashtanga transformative?

BBB: Thom was rigid physically. He was tight physically from his running and his focus on his running. Thom has been doing his practice since 1982. He's Gumby compared to where he started. There's a psychological component to that kind of physical opening. The results have been tremendous psychological growth and overcoming fear.

It's an interesting phenomenon. There is no question that there is a psychological and a spiritual polishing to this practice. In other words, as you become more proficient in the postures, there is a spiritual development. There is also a spiritual entrapment, as you become more efficient. You're opening, you're opening, you're opening, but psychologically you're looking at yourself and saying, "Look how open I'm becoming! Isn't that wonderful! Look at me! Look how flexible! I can put both feet behind my head!"

Because the *ashtanga* practice is such a strong and powerful physical practice, there can be a subtle arrogance that goes with it. But that is true about any spiritual development. Anytime you start to develop the *siddhis*, or the powers, the traps of the ego become more and more subtle. There are some outrageous falls once you start getting past certain points in your spiritual development.

How does one avoid the pitfalls?

BBB: Very good question. Watching. I learned a practice from the Jains called *upa* yoga, which is the yoga of constant vigilance. You are constantly watching yourself and your thoughts.

What has been the fruit of your ashtanga practice?

TB: It opened me up to a deeper compassion and a deeper understanding—first of myself, then of other people. It opened me
up to my greater potential and greater Self.

I have seen great teachers that don't do any practice, and
I have seen great practitioners who are not good teachers.
The practice has taught me how to become a teacher and
how to open up myself to people. In order to be a yoga
teacher, I have to be open and accepting. It's not always easy,
and I am not always on the mark, but yoga has taught me to
be more open and accepting of different people, and things
that I am not used to.

BBB: Here's a good example. Recently we were driving from East
Hampton to New York City. We came through the midtown
tunnel, and just as we broke through the tunnel we see a
woman on the side of the road, hanging her head out of her
BMW and throwing up. An armored car pulls over in front
of her. A guy jumps out, and he's in a uniform. I look at her
and think, "At least she knows these armored car guys aren't
going to rip her off." I said, "Thom, we better stop." So we
pull over behind the armored truck, and I get out. Traffic is
now going around us. A police car comes. We're not a hundred yards out of the tunnel.

TB: This is one of the most highly dense traffic spaces in New
York City.

BBB: Midtown tunnel. Rush hour. Eight-thirty.

TB: Rush hour. Major rush hour.

BBB: So she said, "I can't move! I can't move!" She's having cold sweats. I said, "Look, you've got to move, you can't stay here. We have to get you out of here. These guys in the armored car are going to call an ambulance. Let me drive you around the corner to our apartment, which is four blocks from here. It's on a side street, it's quiet, and it's tree-lined. The air is better. You can sit there and not have hundreds of thousands of people passing you while you're throwing up. You can use our phone. We'll get you water. We'll call your husband on your cell phone."

I said to Thom, "I'll drive her car." So now we're with her. I thought, "Let's get her in a safer spot." She was talking to her friend who had called on her cell phone. I gave her friend the address of our apartment. I said, "We'll meet you there." I'm holding her head as she's throwing up.

Thom has always been very compassionate and sensitive to people, but he also has always had a little bit of xenophobia, a fear of strangers. He was very sheltered and shy and introverted. In his neighborhood where he grew up, you didn't trust strangers.

We get back to our apartment, and I have to leave for an appointment. I have already told this woman, "Come up to our apartment, take a shower, lie down, call your husband, make yourself at home." So Thom is left with this woman and her friend in our apartment. I put these complete strangers in our apartment, and Thom was completely at ease with the situation.

TB: Listen to this note she wrote us: "Dear Thom and Beryl, thank you very much for all that you did. Kindness like this in not common in the nineties, but please know it is appreciated." That really touched me. It taught me to be more compassionate and to act on it.

Beryl Bender Birch graduated from Syracuse University with a degree in philosophy and comparative religion. She is the author of *Power Yoga*, and has been studying and teaching the classical *astanga* yoga path and practice since 1974. She is the founder and co-director of The Hard & The Soft Astanga Yoga Institute in New York City and the Wellness Director of the prestigious New York Road Runners Club. Best known for her work in bringing *astanga* yoga to mainstream America and the traditional athletic community, she has taught her Power Yoga system to thousands of students and athletes.

Thom Birch is co-director of The Hard & The Soft Astanga Yoga Institute in New York City. He holds a B.A. degree in humanistic psychology from the University of Houston. He attended college on a full athletic scholarship and was a track and field All-American. Thom began practicing classical *astanga* yoga in 1982 in order to heal an achilles tendon injury sustained while competing as a professional long distance runner. He has been practicing yoga and running ever since. Thom began teaching with his wife Beryl in 1984, and has since shared his knowledge of yoga and sports with thousands of students and fellow athletes.

Thom and Beryl reside with their three Siberian huskies, Anna, Snowflake, and Hopi in East Hampton, New York.

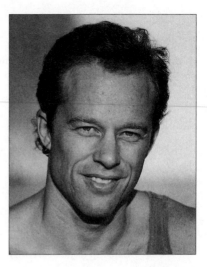

ROD STRYKER
LOS ANGELES

How were you introduced to yoga?

I had a mystical and practical introduction.

First the mystical. I was five. I remember that period of time because it was significant—it was the summer I learned to ride a two-wheeler. I was staying at my granduncle's house. One day, I was looking at a wall of books. I went over and pulled a book off the shelf by chance. I opened it up and it was a book of yoga. I saw this yogi in hundreds of postures. I made a connection to these images of this man and can remember deciding I was going to do that someday.

Wind the tape forward fourteen years. I was nineteen. That's when I started practicing yoga. I had quit school in the middle of my junior year of college, and I was working full-time doing a lot of double shifts. It was the first time I was making a living and really becoming responsible for myself. I showed up to an employee meeting tired. A woman turned to me and said, "You look tired. You should try yoga." I was working so much I could not get to class. She recommended *Light on Yoga* by B.K.S. Iyengar. I read the introduction and was deeply stirred.

Was it the same book you discovered as a child?

Oddly enough, yes, which I believe was fate and a sense of being guided.

Did it occur to you that you had been reintroduced to the same book fourteen years later?

No. I was twenty-four when I realized *Light on Yoga* was the book I picked up when I was nineteen, which was the same book I saw when I was five. I was at the Bodhi Tree looking at yoga books, and I came across *Light on Yoga*. Suddenly, I had the image of being five and seeing the same postures.

Was the recognition a powerful experience?

I marveled at it. I have only brought it up in conversation to a few people in my life, but it is significant. It's a sense of being led. Through experiences like that I was left with a sense of wonder. But just as significant to me is my first word as a child. It wasn't "mom" or "dad," it was "light," so I think I was a yogi from the beginning.

I was doing *asanas* out of *Light on Yoga*. The second or third pose that I did was *parsvakonasana*. I held it a minute or two and started breaking out into a sweat. I had been athletic all my life, and to have such an immediate experience with something so dynamic, and yet so static, was very provocative. It was very evocative, and I immediately felt benefits from it.

The benefits were manifesting in my work, my energy level, and my sleep. It was a trying time in terms of my emotional and psychological development. I had quit school and had reached some dead ends in terms of my lifestyle. I wasn't very grounded. I didn't have a sense of where I was going. I knew I had to change friends, but I didn't know how. Yoga immediately became an anchor for me. It wasn't long before I started practicing every day for an hour and feeling tremendous shifts in my life.

Did you have a strong desire to teach or was it a gradual process?

It was much more *vinyasa krama*, which means intelligent or wise progression. I first spent nine months doing *Light on Yoga* quite committedly. I moved back to Los Angeles, and a friend of mine, who had just started *kundalini* yoga a week or two earlier, took me to my first class. I practiced *kundalini* yoga for about two years. It was good for me, but not particularly balanced as I look back.

I had gotten very serious about my yoga practice, when I met a girl who introduced me to Alan Finger. At first, I didn't like Alan's class, because I didn't feel it was serious enough. It felt a little too light and I couldn't relate to it, but a few weeks later I went back. The thing that spun it in a new direction was that I sat with him privately. In the system that he's from and that I learned, the hub of one's yoga practice is meeting with a teacher. The practice of yoga is traditionally and most powerfully sourced by having one-on-one contact with a teacher/master and then a personal practice based on that.

I met with Alan about six weeks after participating in his group classes. He gave me a couple of meditation techniques and my own practice suited for my needs. I remember sitting down alone and doing this practice, and it really felt like I was taking an adventure into spirit. I really didn't know why I was doing it, but I had enough faith, and I did it. Over the next three months, I began to feel real shifts in my personality, in my understanding of myself, and in my sense of Self.

I had been doing yoga for three years, and with Alan for six months, when it dawned on me to approach Alan, which I did the next time I had a private with him. I said, "I would like to teach." It was really just a sense of wanting to know more. That's why I wanted to teach. He said, "Oh, very good, I told my wife that you were the first American who I wanted to study under me, but I wanted you to approach me. I have been waiting for you to do that," which was very wise on his part. He said, "Here's a teaching *mantra* to initiate you and in two weeks you're teaching." I said, "Wait a second! I don't know if I want to teach quite that fast, maybe we could slow down the snowball!" My aspirations in the beginning were fairly low-key. I wanted to get deeper into yoga. I didn't want to make a living from teaching. That was the last thing that dawned on me. I was interested in being an actor.

When did you make the transition from being an actor to being a yoga teacher?

There was an odd little arc to the whole thing. I was very committed to being an actor. I was going to class, auditions, and doing all the busyness that actors have to do. I was making a living exclusively from teaching yoga for several years at this point. To be honest with you, I can't imagine how I did both. The interesting thing was that the height of when I worked as an actor was the beginning of its end, though not voluntarily.

There a saying from the *Old Testament*: "Man proposes and the universe disposes." If I had made a proposal to the universe it would have been "Let me succeed as an actor and always be a yogi." And eventually I did. I had been teaching *Ishta* yoga for six years when I got a part on a soap and a three-year contract, which is a great thing for an actor. I really thought I was saying good-bye to making a living as a teacher. However, between getting the job and going to work, CBS decided to cancel the show. I only got to do one month, but I had a great time actually.

There was no big deal afterward. I was just another actor looking for a job. The next year I didn't really work, and it was a pretty frustrating time. It finally occurred to me that teaching yoga was incredibly profound—I just didn't make as much money as successful actors. When I taught, I was in a creative zenith, and then I would pull myself out of the zenith to go try and act. The disparity between thriving as a teacher and then scraping together as an actor eventually was the final straw.

When I speak of acting, I feel like I'm talking about somebody else. I don't have any connection to it at all. We think we want things and the universe doesn't necessarily give us those things, but it will give us the feelings we want to have if we had those things. That's my experience.

You recently went from yoga teacher to yoga studio owner. What was your motivation for the transition?

Varied. There are a lot of things I could mention. Certainly there was a financial element, but that's not the main one. Something is lacking in the whole preparation for teachers in the United States right now. I would like to build something better, something more significant, and teach from my own conviction, teach from my own heart. It's important stuff. It's one of the few legacies you have as a yoga teacher.

When you create a studio, you leave class and you've got product. The product as a yoga teacher is that you are making people feel different. You are hopefully making them feel better. And perhaps teaching people how to make people feel better, as well. Maybe you make a video, and you've got something for future generations to take a look at, but mostly what we do as teachers is pretty intangible. I feel committed to doing what is unique to my vision of yoga and my experience with yoga.

What is your definition of spirituality?

When we say the word "spiritual," I'm frightened of people's interpretation, because we all have this vague sense of what spiritual is. I don't think it only means meditating. There are plenty of people who are meditating and are not spiritually awake. I don't think any methodology necessarily guarantees spirituality.

Spirituality is an expansiveness and the freedom to express one's Self in life completely. It is not just an experience either. It means living in accord with universal principles of fairness and integrity. It is being vibrant and alive in one's emotional life, as one is in one's creative life. As one is in one's creative life, as one is in one's devotional life. As one is in one's devotional life, as one is in one's business life. In short, it is giving more than you take. Leaving the world in some way better by your actions.

Just because you can get into *eka pada sirsasana*, it's no guarantee of really being fully alive. Mani Finger says, "Yoga means life. Yoga means living." It's really the science of how to be fully alive. That's what spirituality means to me. Knowing what day of the week it is. Knowing there is suffering on the other end of town. It's not closing our eyes to political or sociological issues. Knowing we exist as psychological beings, as well as spiritual beings, as well as energetic beings. That's what intrigues me about living, and also intrigues me about what the right yoga methods can help to enhance.

How could one have a meditation practice and still remain unenlightened?

For the same reason that when you go to sleep, you wake up and in a few minutes the same neurotic chatter is there. Meditation is just a tool. Are you using the right tool? The Tibetans talk about meditating with a hood on. Just because you're having some experience that doesn't necessarily mean it's waking you up.

It goes back to the theory of yoga and the importance of *tapas*. *Tapas* means "to heat" and "to purify." We all have tendencies. We all come from somewhere, and we all have a momentum going somewhere. Our momentum colors our experiences and what we are attracted to. It is only through the idea of *tapas*, of purification, that we can activate or germinate our hidden potential. For someone who loves to meditate passively, loves to sit and reflect, their *tapas* might be doing active meditation—*kriya, chakras, pranayama,* and *mudras.* That actually might be the most provocative, beneficial.

Changing people's momentum gives them an opportunity to reflect more than if they just continued in the same momentum. Desikachar says, "If someone loves to read and study *sutras*, or yoga philosophy, and that's what they feel compelled to do, but practice is something they are not very attracted to, put them in a practice and it could actually inform them much more than those books could." It's the idea of doing something different than we are attracted to do. That's going to have more impact in getting us to wake up. Some people love static postures. Put them in a movement class. They may not like it, but what we like and what we need to become more aware is rarely the same thing.

What is the key to a balanced practice?

The key is a teacher. You've got to have a teacher. I had two very powerful teachers who came from a very holistic understanding of yoga. Alan's father, Mani, was taught by some of the most powerful yogis of this century—Paramahansa Yogananda, Swami Sivananda, Venkatesananda, and Bharati, who was called the Shakespeare of India and was a *Tantric* hermit. He lived alone in a cave in the Himalayas for eighteen years.

Once you have had a certain amount of time in a tradition, you still need a guru. You still need someone who reflects to you who you are. The way yoga thrives in America is very unique in the yoga paradigm. Typically, American discipleship is either too dependent, where we rely on the guru to fulfill our emotional needs, or too independent. We don't want anyone in our life who might examine us deeply at our core, beyond even the facility of a therapist. So we take group classes. We take a little bit from this teacher. We take some from that teacher. A new workshop teacher comes into town, and we take from them. We go on a retreat with a different teacher. The problem is that we keep learning from teachers who were never really steeped in a tradition with a single teacher. Or we're working with teachers who never worked with a teacher who had a holistic understanding of all of yoga, who were masters.

The best case scenario is that you have a teacher/master who can give you all of those things. If you look at the popular teachers who we revere the most, whether it's Iyengar, Pattabhi Jois, Desikachar, Sivananda, Krishnamacharya, Swami Satchidananda, or Yogananda, all of those teachers came from a *mula* tradition, which means they had a root. They steeped themselves with one teacher—a master. The teachers I just named are by far some of the most influential, and yet we're setting this watered-down precedent where typically we're studying with teachers who have studied with a lot of different teachers, and mostly the emphasis is on the body, not the soul.

An old metaphor I read from Vivekananda said, "The student becomes like the man, who looking for water, digs many shallow holes and never strikes water." That's my concern about modern-day yoga discipleship in the United States. My experience is that when you do work with a teacher who has more depth, and the ability to disseminate and transmit to you as an individual for your specific needs, the possibility of what you can gain is ten-fold from just going out and doing more physical practices.

But the Indian yogis you mentioned come from a guru-based culture.

You bring up a good point. The challenge is that we have a different relationship to relationship. In the Indian culture where yoga was born, there is a culture of devotion, a culture of surrender. In America, it's a culture of psychology. It's a culture of intellectual understanding. There is a trust implicit in the Indian culture that allows for more balance.

In America, mentorship suffers. It doesn't have to be a spiritual tradition. An apprentice studied with a blacksmith, but he didn't only go for blacksmith technology. He saw what it was like to be a man around a blacksmith. He saw how the guy ate. He saw how the guy related to his wife. He saw how the guy showed up. Through storytelling, the blacksmith forged a lot of different stories about life. The apprentice saw suffering and pleasure through the mentor. That also doesn't exist in America.

Lack of mentorship is part of the problem. I was taught that the teacher should be careful of who he picks as a student. The student should be as careful as the teacher is. You should only have faith in the teacher to the degree in which your work with him verifies your trust. It is my opinion that there are very few teachers worth fully committing to. I was very lucky. I was led to teachers who are human beings and still have foibles. But there was no agenda about trying to take advantage of me or delude me in any way for their own advancement or their own power. They had tremendous power, technology, and understanding. That was a gift. They gave that gift to me. I will always be grateful.

It is a chain. There is an aspect of this that really defies rationale. In the teachings, there is also transmission. By transmission, I mean there is presence shared from the teacher to the taught. If you are only getting technology from your teacher, something is missing.

There is a relationship of transmission if your transformation is to be lasting. You will be imparted something that is beyond words and beyond technique. Through my lineage, I am hooked up to a hermit sitting in a cave several hundred years ago who sat and sat and sat, and delved into the mystery of his own spiritual being and reached tremendous realization. Through transmission, that experience has been handed down.

We think of technology in terms of microchips and moon shots. What is your definition of technology?

I mean a tool. What distinguishes yoga from religion is the difference between science and belief. Scientifically, we have proof. We can show you that if you inhale through your left nostril it creates a response in your right brain. That's a technology. A hammer is technology. A screwdriver is technology. They are both tools, and yet both have very different applications. The yoga context is, "When do I want to lengthen exhale relative to inhale? When should I lengthen inhale relative to exhale?" Well, one's a screwdriver and one's a hammer.

It this day and age, you don't need a religious belief. Acupuncture, for instance, is not based on religion. You don't need any belief for acupuncture to work. Stick the needle in, and it's going to change or influence the pathways of energy in your system. It's going to have an effect. When acupuncture first came to America, it was considered a religion. It was illegal. Then they discovered all of these world-class athletes were getting their injuries needled, and they were healing much faster. The athletes weren't Taoists. Yoga is the same thing. It doesn't require a belief.

Faith is not the same thing as belief. I have faith, and it has always been very alive. I think that is incredibly important. The tremendous benefits and profound changes I have enjoyed because of yoga have, I believe, hinged on my faith that it could work. There is a beautiful teaching in Sogyal Rinpoche's *The Tibetan Book of Living and Dying*. He talks about a specific *mantra* that is a very profound and central in the Tibetan tradition. It says that to the degree to which one feels pain or disconnection or suffering, one should apply an equal amount of that same longing and intensity into accepting divine presence. When we are not feeling whole or complete, if we can turn that inside out and say with that same intensity, "I do feel a connection, there is a connection," it can be lifted, and it can be transformed. That's faith.

Since you spoke of technology as tools, what are the nuts and bolts of your personal practice and meditation?

My practice revolves around meditation. The hub of the wheel is ultimately the vehicle of silence. The word in Sanskrit is *kaivalya*. It means "without coloring" or "aloneness." The last chapter in Patajali's *Yoga Sutras* is called *Kaivalyapadah*. It is linked to liberation or being free. That is what my practice is an inspiration towards every day. Sitting to me is automatic. Practice varies with the different phases of life. Some phases of life are more challenging intellectually. Some are more challenging physically. Some are more taxing creatively. The practices I do will vary depending upon what is happening in my life.

The methodology of pairing a practice with one's individual needs is called *Anava-upaya* yoga. I have been teaching *Ishta* yoga for seventeen years. It took me eight or nine years before I could do that for myself. I used to get different techniques from my teachers, and I would do those techniques for three months, to six months, to nine months. When I was in my early twenties, I worked pretty hard on *asanas*, but it still was in conjunction with meditation. I don't work that hard. My body changed. I have an advanced practice, but the poses came because I was meditating and doing *pranayama*, and the deeper energetic practices of *Tantra* and *Kriya* yogas. My body got softer and became willing to meld into the postures, because I was doing the other deeper work. I am convinced of that.

There is a Sanskrit word *kriyavati* in the *Hatha Yoga Pradipika*, which is our oldest book of hatha yoga. *Kriyavati* refers to a state of being where you are flowing into the postures effortlessly. They are on a very advanced level, and yet you're not working hard. You're linked up to a deeper realm, a deeper level. Do I feel that all the time? Absolutely not. But there have been practices of *kriyavati* that came out of the energetic condition that I evoked when meditating. That facilitated openings and breakthroughs in my body that might have taken me much longer if I was just working hard physically, because the yoga was working on a deeper level. Those experiences have colored and affected my body years later.

My personal approach is to do a balanced routine with subtle differences in the emphasis every day. I create emphasis on what I need. This morning I knew I had a very long and demanding day, so it was headstand, because headstand is more energetic than shoulderstand. I didn't do shoulderstand today. I did postures that would combine well with headstand. I don't spend as much time doing *asanas* as I used to. For a long time, it was about an hour of meditation and *pranayama*, and an hour-and-a-half of *asanas* a day. Now it's about forty-five minutes and an hour, or forty-five minutes and a half-hour.

Do you start with meditation?

I do.

Why?

The meditations that I do are more active. I am not just sitting and watching, so it requires more attention. The mind is more alert at the beginning of the practice than at the end of the practice, although it may feel a little dull if it's early morning. I do a few movements just to start things rolling, but I don't spend a lot of time doing postures, because it allows me to really get in there and work with my mind. If you're doing a lot of *asana* before you work on meditation, your mind is a blank because you've opened yourself and you've released all that tension. It's a little more interesting and provocative to sit down and deal with your mind in meditation, rather than wiping it out in postures. Then the postures help me iron out the creases of tension or inhibition or stress that I haven't reached through meditation. Also, the postures afterwards are more grounding.

Is that specific to the Ishta tradition?

Ishta says some people need it one way, some people need another. If I find someone who is extremely tense and there is no way they can sit still, clearly they need to do postures and breathing before they meditate. But we are not dependent on the *asana* to provide a relaxed enough state of mind to get us into that meditative state.

What is the fruit of meditation?

Only through meditation can I access a state of aliveness and purity on an energetic, psychological, emotional, spiritual, and physical level. The *Hatha Yoga Pradipika* says that when *siddhasana* is mastered, what need is there for any of the other poses? When you have that, there's no need for all the other *asanas*. The body is simply a data bank for the mind. If you clean your mind, if your mind is relaxed, your body needs less *asana*. Once you have a certain degree of equanimity, there is no need to keep pounding away at your body. The treasure is inside. The treasure is actually happening effortlessly in every moment. It's not something that's years and years away. You don't have to spend thirteen years mastering *asanas* before you find it.

There is a pristine place in each of us that is of the same stuff that lights the most distant star. It is life itself. It is destiny and all the levels of creation happening at once. *Now.* I recognize it and I am reminded of the truth, of what is real, of what is essential. That is the fruit of meditation.

Rod Stryker began practicing yoga at the age of nineteen. He started teaching in 1980, soon after beginning his apprenticeship with Yogiraj Alan Finger and Alan's father and yoga master, Mani Finger. Fifteen years later, his teachers gave him the title of master in their school of Tantra Yoga. Rod has produced or appeared in three award-winning *New Yoga* videos with fitness guru Kathy Smith.

Rod was married in May of 1998. He lives in Los Angeles with his wife, Cheryl; step-son, Zack; their dogs, Olive and Tara; and Cutie Pie, their guinea pig.

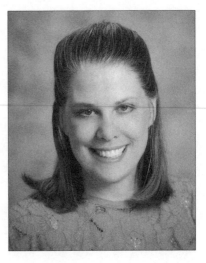

RAMA BERCH

SAN DIEGO

What is the key to yoga?

It has to be alive. It has to be experienced. I was talking to someone recently who has been studying Patanjali's *Yoga Sutras* and is getting very analytical about the whole process. The way this teacher was describing it sounded like another list of "shoulds." "I should do this, and I should do that. I should think this way and I should think that way." We already have enough of those. I teach the *Yoga Sutras*, and the other texts that I work with, as if they were car manuals. How do you change the air filter on the carburetor? How do you unlock the glove box? Not "you should do it this way," but "it works when you do it this way." If you approach the *sutras* like they are asking you questions, you will look at your experience.

When you have an experience, then you have yoga.

You can have the experience by looking at the stars or watching the sunset. And that for me is yoga. You have to realize that it's not in the technique. Whatever technique you have is a catalyst for getting into the experience. *Asanas* can be used that way, but *asanas* in and of themselves are not yoga. If *asanas* are done with merely the emphasis on the physical perfection, they look like a form of gymnastics. The best gymnasts in the world are thirteen-year-old girls. I'm not going to be thirteen again in this lifetime, and you were never a girl. How good are you going to be at some of those moves? If you spend your whole life trying to perfect them, what have you got? The point is to get to that experience. When you are completely present in the moment, then you are living in that incredible state of awareness.

If you have never eaten a chocolate-covered strawberry, anything I try to tell you about that experience is going to be incomplete. I can say, "Chocolate is creamy." And you might say, "Oh, is it like pudding?" I could say, "No. Chocolate is sweet." And you might say, "Oh, is it like sugar?" "No, it's creamy *and* sweet." I can say a whole list of words, but they will never really describe what the experience is like. How do you tell someone what it's like? You give them a chocolate-covered strawberry and they go, 'Ah.'"

In the *Yoga Sutras*, Patanjali says the exact description of this experience is what a dumb man, meaning one who cannot speak, says when he tastes something sweet for the first time. He can say nothing. There are many texts that give beautiful descriptions of this experience, and they still don't do it justice.

What causes inflexibility?

There are usually a lot of reasons for the body to be tight. People talk about emotions being locked up in the body. I think that's both true and untrue. Some people will vividly recall a memory when you open up a spot around their spine or heart area, or you free up their neck for the first time, or they get movement in a hip, or they find a new way to stand. It's like they are reliving the experience. They may have a wave of emotion. They may have tears or anger, cry out in anguish, or pound the floor.

You may have had a series of unpleasant childhood experiences, and the way you got through them was by holding your breath and locking up your back. Since then you've sorted out all the emotional stuff, but you're still holding your breath and your back is still locked. You haven't re-patterned the body. You may not have any memory associated with it at all, because you've already let go of it.

There's another possibility. Let's say you didn't have any bad childhood experiences, not that anybody fits into that category! Let's say you had a wonderful childhood, but your mother walked with a little bit of a limp, because when she was fourteen, she fell off a horse and broke her leg. You learned to walk by watching your mother. No one ever pointed out to you that you walked with a little bit of a limp. You may have learned body patterns that don't relate to any experience you had at all, and you need to re-pattern. There may have been nothing to process.

This is not an exhaustive list of why your body is the way it is. There can be so many reasons the body is locked up. It isn't necessarily locked up emotions. With yoga, you don't have to necessarily dig up all the reasons. Psychotherapy is a different process. There can be value in recognizing and understanding what influenced the way you are, but yoga is letting go of that.

Here's an example. Have you ever had a storage shed? They're awful.

They're full.

They're full, but do you know what's in the storage shed?

No idea.

I had this storage shed for about two years, and every month I would write the rent check. It would disturb me, because I was writing a rent check for a storage shed, and I didn't even know what was in it anymore. The thought of renting a truck, going over there, digging all of the stuff out, looking through the boxes, figuring out what to do with it—whether to keep it, give it away, have a garage sale, take it to the swap meet, or give it to friends—was so bad that I would just mail the rent check. The next month, I would go through the whole process again.

One day, I rented a truck. I took the boxes unopened and put them in the back of the truck. I drove to the dump and pushed the boxes out. To this day I don't know what I got rid of, but I haven't missed it. If I hadn't needed it in two years, I wasn't going to need it again. Maybe I threw away some good stuff, but that was all I could handle at that point in time. It's a great metaphor for yoga. Just let it go. You don't have to pull it all out of the boxes and figure it all out. You can just toss it. Who are you if you don't own all that stuff? Yoga says you're free.

How did you come to the tradition of yoga?

I became interested in yoga by seeing photos and articles in women's magazines when I was a mother with three young children in the early seventies. Then I started doing yoga with Richard Hittleman and Lilias Folan when their shows came on TV. I consider them my first two yoga teachers. Eventually I bought a yoga book. I was an off-again, on-again yogi. I never even went to a yoga class. I had an interest in yoga, but it didn't seem to capture me. In retrospect, I was really an excellent candidate for being a couch potato. I had no interest in exercise or movement. My hands were full as a mom, and I was pursuing a career in management.

In the mid-seventies, I encountered a meditation teacher and had an extraordinary meditation experience. Each day I would sit and meditate as I had been taught. As I would sit to meditate, the energy moving through my body, which is called *kundalini*, would move me into spontaneous yoga postures—positions I could never get into if I were trying. I recognized them as being yoga poses. This really accelerated my interest in the physical practice. I went to a few yoga classes, and they were teaching the yoga poses differently than what I was experiencing in meditation. I would sit for an hour of meditation and move continuously, and at the same time get deeper and deeper levels of meditative state. Things were being opened and healed in my body that I didn't even know were problems. Then I would go to a yoga class, and it was very different. It was almost artificial.

I began looking for more training in hatha yoga, so I took a teacher training. I started teaching, but what I was teaching didn't match what I was getting in meditation, so I took another teacher training. In total, I have received training in four traditions. Each of them taught me to do the poses as though I were doing something.

In 1983, I had a serious injury in a traffic accident. Another car hit my car head-on. My injuries were soft tissue damage, but I was in constant, agonizing pain. I was in bed for six months, and I could not do the yoga poses the way I been taught. I couldn't sit to meditate. I could only get up for short periods of time. I began with breathing and little movements. I began to reconstruct, through my own exploration of my body with the principles of the yoga practice, what I had been shown for almost ten years. I had the help of a lot of loving and wonderful people—chiropractors, massage therapists, healers, psychics. I learned and received healing from all of them.

After six months, I became physically functional again. I went from being active two hours a day to being active six or eight hours a day. It took me almost two years to get back to where I could run what most people consider a normal schedule. Then I had another traffic accident. This time a truck bounced off the side of my car and threw me into the fast lane on the freeway headed the wrong direction. Amazingly, there was a gap in the traffic, and I was able to back off to the side of the road. That was certainly symbolic—I was headed the wrong direction in life.

My body was beat up soft tissue-wise again. I went home and I started breathing. I started exploring deep levels of musculature and tissue in the body millimeter by millimeter. I never missed a day of work. I never spent a day in bed. It took me about three months to go through that reconstruction process. I did get some medical care. There are times in our life where we need medical care, and I heartily support anyone who is getting that.

I was still teaching the way I had been taught to teach. The discrepancy between my personal practice and teaching became more and more uncomfortable for me. Teaching became a situation in which I was not living my life with integrity. I began sneaking little things into the classes. I call it "sneaky yoga." Students started having extraordinary changes in their bodies. Over a period of time, I came to trust that what I was doing really did open the body from the inside out, really was replicating what I had been given by the extraordinary gift of initiation from a great master. The way that I teach is an outgrowth of that exploration.

About four years ago, Vyaas Houston suggested that we give this style of yoga a name. He said, "If you don't give it a name, they're going to call it Rama yoga," which was not going to be okay with me. We went through appropriate names and selected the name *Svaroopa* yoga. *Svaroopa* means "the bliss of the Self." We use the poses as a means of getting people into the foundation of consciousness, but along the way, the poses are incredibly supportive to the healing and transformation process. The deeper awareness of our own being is always there. We're just looking in the other direction. One master says, "It's the bliss that rages continually." As soon as the mind becomes quiet, the bliss of your own being bursts forth spontaneously.

Is the goal of Svaroopa *yoga to experience* kundalini?

While I have been very fortunate to have that as a key factor in my entire path, I don't think it's essential for people to get *kundalini* awakening. I see many people getting tremendous benefit from yoga practice, whether their *kundalini* awakens or not. And not just from this style of yoga—all styles of yoga. In some students that we work with, *kundalini* begins to move, and in some of them, it doesn't. But every student that we work with, their spine begins to move, their breath opens up, their aches and pains go away, their mind becomes more peaceful, and their life begins to change. Most yoga teachers can say that. It's one of the most wonderful things about yoga.

Have you come to view your car accidents as non-accidents?

Someone once told me that the definition of coincidence is God's way of remaining anonymous. I would put them in that category. In one, I was headed in one direction and someone ran straight into the front end of my car. "You're not going this way." In the other, I was headed down the freeway, and someone put me headed the wrong direction in the fast lane. "You're not going this way anymore." Each one was a divinely ordained experience to force me to look at what I knew, instead of relying on what I had been taught. To look at my own experience and to trust it and to teach from it, instead of drawing on other people's words and other people's experiences. I would call them messages from God, but it took a big message for me to get it.

Where were you living before San Diego?

I spent about fifteen years on the road. There were a couple of times I settled down and stayed in one place, but I basically lived out of the suitcase, moving from one city to another, *ashram* to *ashram*. Sometimes I would stay in a city, work for a while, make some money, and then live on it for awhile in various *ashrams*. The travel started with the meditation experience that I had. I knew it was what I had been looking for all my life. I sold my business and my house, and I went to India to live with my guru. I raised my three children in the *ashram*. As he would move from place to place with the teachings, we would travel and work and study with him.

When I was on the road, I would go to various temples of longitude. In Europe, I would go to the cathedrals. In Japan and China, I would go to the temples and mosques. I vividly remember standing in one of the most beautiful mosques, the National Mosque of Malaysia. I had been to mosques before, and I could not feel that rich, deeper layer of existence, so I kept returning. I was standing in the women's corner, and I got it. It was the last one for me. I had been to all of the various religions and traditions. I had spent fifteen years temple hopping. When I got that one, I didn't need to go anymore. I needed to find it in every place. Then I discovered I didn't need to go anyplace. After that, I settled in San Diego.

Your yoga center offers yoga therapy. Would it be wise for this to be covered by insurance?

Would it be wise? I can say, "Yes," and I can say, "No." Let me weave my way around these. We have a physician associated with

Master Yoga, who sees the value of yoga and yoga therapy. He has been supervising and treating patients with yoga and yoga therapy, and getting amazing results. He has done research and gives a very wonderful presentation explaining why yoga and yoga therapy can work to reduce pain and promote healing. With his involvement, we have been able to treat a number of people under their medical insurance, so I am not answering from the theoretical point of view. Physicians in California can supervise any kind of therapy, as long as it doesn't cost too much money and the patient gets better. It's to the insurance company's advantage for the patient to get better. Yoga can be billed as a certain type of physical therapy, which it is. If you go to physical therapists, you get a lot of yoga poses.

We have found two distinctly different types of results. One is that the patient has a prescription for six to twelve weeks of yoga therapy. They come every week, learn a little yoga, get fantastically better, start to do yoga on their own, and we never see them again. Success. They understand that they have to do something to provide for the continued care of their own body. Then we have a different kind of person entirely. They come in for a session of yoga therapy, feel better, go back home, start to hurt, and start to complain again. They never come back. They don't want to do anything for themselves. They want someone else to make them feel better. They don't want to do yoga therapy. They want to go have a massage. When they have a massage, they lay there and someone else makes them feel better. When they do yoga therapy, they have to move, breathe, answer questions, look at their emotions, and take responsibility for doing yoga on their own.

We have had people under medical insurance who don't come back. We have people who pay for their therapy and come again and again. It's not a matter of who pays for it. It's a matter of who feels responsible.

The medical world is very interested in therapies that used to be called alternative or holistic health. The phraseology is very important. In the last two years, the medical profession has called it complementary medicine. Now they are moving toward a new phrase—integrated medicine. They are very interested in bringing other modalities into what we call traditional Western medicine. They recognize they are not able to help all patients. Doctors have a bad name is this country. I find them to be incredibly caring people who want to be healers and don't know how. Every doctor I know lives with a great deal of frustration when they have patients they can't help.

A study published in the *New England Journal of Medicine* said that a third of the American population had visited holistic or alternative health practitioners in the preceding year. They spent more money visiting holistic practitioners than they spent visiting doctors. More people are going in for alternative or complementary care. Yoga falls in that category. More people are taking responsibility and spending time and money to preserve a state of health, rather than to allow themselves to fall into a condition of disease and pain.

What is your opinion concerning national standards for yoga teachers?

It's an important issue because yoga is becoming such a strong river of consciousness. I have lived with that question for over two years, and I have been on both sides of it—yea and nay. There is wide variety in styles. There is extremely wide diversity in the training a person can get before they teach. Certain teacher training programs will train you to be a teacher in a weekend. Our teacher training program is five hundred hours. A lot of teachers have never taken a teacher training program, but they started teaching because they were doing yoga, and they loved it. One thing I have found—the number of people who get hurt is extraordinarily small. Most people who get hurt in yoga classes hurt themselves. The teacher doesn't hurt them. Even with a very strenuous, physically demanding approach, it's amazing how few people get hurt. You can't say that about the gym. You can't say that about jogging. There is a tremendous safety zone in yoga. Because of that, for a long time I objected to the idea of creating standards. Yoga traditionally has not been about external standards at all. If the teacher is bad, people quit going to them.

Yoga was never designed to treat medical conditions. *Ayurveda* is designed to treat medical conditions, but yoga does do dramatic things for the body, the mind, and the emotions. I have found it to be a tremendous help with my aches and pains. I have been very fortunate to work with people in terms of giving them their body back and giving them their life back. Yoga is now gaining the reputation as being a form of complementary medicine. When we have yoga teachers prescribing and treating for conditions, we must have a standard of training and background. Standards have been set up in Europe. We need to set up standards for the training of yoga teachers and the certification of yoga teachers, and it's a very touchy subject. I call it the yoga of the yoga teachers. If the yoga teachers can't come together in union, who's going to be able to?

What does your personal practice consist of?

I am always in a yoga pose. If I'm standing, I'm in *tadasana*. If I'm sitting, I'm in *virasana*. If you're in a body, you're in *asana*. Either a good one, or a bad one. You're either in *asana* that's opening up and taking care of your body, or you're in one that's closing up and bringing your body downhill. *Asana* is simply body position.

I do asana practice in the morning and in the evening. It depends on how much my body needs. I will go through time periods where I'm focusing on a particular type of practice. I will be doing strong standing poses or a lot of abdominal work. Then I will go through another period where I'm just doing long, deep, slow twists. Where I'm at and what I need changes over time. The amount of physical practice also varies. Depending on what the challenges are for the day, I will practice anywhere from ten minutes to three hours in the morning. In the evening, I usually do forty-five minutes. I also do a breathing practice before I go to sleep, because it's very soothing to my nervous system.

I consistently do three hours of meditation, no matter what. Because the practices that I do, I spend very little time sleeping compared to the normal person. I prefer to spend time at a deeper level of consciousness. My practice is primarily meditation. Through meditation, I can clear and open my body faster than through *asana*. When you start living in your body more, the amount of *asana* you need as a concentrated practice diminishes greatly.

What have you learned from your travels?

It isn't particularly what we need to draw from other cultures. We need to look at what spans through all the cultures. In every culture, there is a place for love. In every culture, there is a place for family. In every culture, there is a place for commitment. In every culture, there is a place for the highest and best principles of human life.

When I traveled, my favorite thing to do, besides temple hopping, was to play bus roulette. You get on a bus that you don't where it's going. Then you get off when you don't know where you are, preferably in a city or countryside where you don't speak the language. And there you are. I would go to these countries and intentionally get lost, so that I could lose myself. Part of myself that I wanted to lose was heavy. It was my negativity, my fears, my resistance, and my old ideas of who I am. I didn't have any of those props for an identity. I would stand there in that incredible newness and delight of just being. Not being anything or being anyone, just being. I would have the most extraordinary encounters with people without having any words get in the way. I always found my way home again.

I didn't learn a lot about the cultures. I learned that everybody has a heart, and the most unlikely people would be welcoming and helpful.

Rama Berch left her successful career as an accountant to undertake training in yoga, meditation, healing, massage, and Eastern traditions. She later moved to India with her three children to study, practice, and live yoga in an *ashram* setting. Rama is the creator and supervisor of the yoga program for Dr. Deepak Chopra's Center for Well Being, as well as founder of Master Yoga Academy in La Jolla, California. She has received certification and training in four schools as a hatha yoga teacher, and is the creator of *Svaroopa* yoga. She teaches extensively in the United States and Canada.

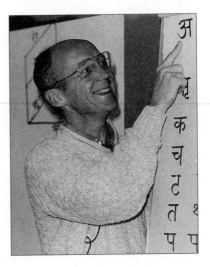

VYAAS HOUSTON
WARWICK, NEW YORK

Why did your life gravitate to Sanskrit?

I love teaching yoga and I love teaching yoga philosophy, but I have a special passion for teaching Sanskrit. It is such a beautiful, exquisite vehicle for sharing sound, knowledge, inspiration, and creativity with other people. It's a very exciting process that requires total focus. It requires heart, soul, mind, and voice.

Yoga mastery is available to anyone who chooses it. It's not the image that I used to have of one powerful yogi sitting isolated by himself, different from other people, which is something that I wanted to be at some point. I see it now as something that anyone can choose. Sanskrit is a great empowerment towards yoga mastery. The aspect of sound and resonance that opens up through the chanting of the language, and the refinement of vibration and sensitivity to vibration that develops from contact with the Sanskrit language is an essential aspect of yoga. It goes hand in hand with meditation, with *asana*, and with developing a practice of being focused. It's as much a part of yoga as the one-pointedness that is required to move on to more advanced yoga postures.

How did you develop the color-coding of the Sanskrit alphabet?

I had started working with computers. After spending all day on the computer, I would sit and meditate at night, and I would see a computer screen. Then I would see diagrams of Sanskrit grammar on the screen in color. I began to see the possibility of color-coding, and I started testing it out on a class. I was amazed at how quickly this group began to understand Sanskrit. They caught fire and this methodology of color-coding the grammar of Sanskrit began to evolve. The more it evolved, the more excited this group got. In fifteen years, I had seen very few people actually put Sanskrit together. Even though my teacher was extraordinary, I noticed that just by method of chanting alone, there were only a handful of people who really began to see how the language worked. Suddenly, I had this group of six people who were putting it all together very rapidly and were tremendously excited about it.

Because of the level of excitement, they began to support each other's learning in a way that I had never seen. Up to that point, I had seen mostly competition in the classes, even with myself. There was always competition. This was the first time I had ever seen a group of people applauding each other's learning. I saw it intensify their learning skills.

It was a quantum leap as far as I was concerned. For fifteen years, I had maybe fifteen students over that entire period of time. Within four years of color-coding the Sanskrit alphabet and changing the whole methodology for accessing the language into a supportive yoga practice, I taught fifteen hundred people.

My teacher used a lot of transliteration. He would use English lettering in addition to the Sanskrit. I didn't know anybody who had achieved any level of depth in Sanskrit through the English letters. Everybody I knew who had really learned Sanskrit was reading the Devanagari script. I took another leap. I cut out transliteration completely and began to teach through the Devanagari script. That was another big breakthrough. It's so much more effective to approach the *sutras* through the Sanskrit language, rather than through English translation. In class, we're getting people to look over and over again at these beautiful, colored letters written in calligraphy. It's been a great way to get people's focus and attention, and to get intimate with the original characters very quickly.

Around the time I developed color-coding, I was beginning to leave the *ashram* environment and set out on my own. I didn't know how I was going to make the transition. I did not have the confidence that I could just teach Sanskrit and be successful enough to support my family. But due to this class, I began to be drawn more just to teaching Sanskrit. To me, it was time to really introduce Sanskrit to the Western world. I decided I would take a big leap of faith. I made a declaration at that point, "I can teach Sanskrit to anybody who wants to learn." I moved to Warwick and created a weekend Sanskrit training. I had no idea if it was going to work, but it caught on and the interest came.

Did the interest arise within the yoga community?

Within the yoga community, and then it began to happen outside the yoga community. I think the most important part was seeing a supportive learning environment. I saw people not competing with each other, but supporting each other and learning. Over the next couple of years, what evolved was a very precise learning model entirely based on the principles of yoga—choosing a point to focus on.

We had agreements within a group that supported people staying focused on the point, even when they obviously would go off the point. One of the agreements was that the class moves on only when everybody gets it. The way we phrase it in the workshop is, "We move on only when I get it." It's because of individuals who have kept that agreement that I have been able to see all the subtle little steps that previously were missing to give people access to Sanskrit. It's not something that requires genius for language, which I never had. It's not necessary to be musical. It is applying the principles of yoga to the pleasure of making sound in the same way we enjoyed making sound when we were small.

When did you begin your journey with yoga?

I started when I was in college in the sixties. I was really searching for something to focus on for the rest of my life, and I wasn't finding it in college, so I was struggling. I was actually concerned about failing out and being drafted to fight in the Vietnam War. I had to go to summer school at the end of my sophomore year to make up a course. I ran into a guy who was an acquaintance of mine, and he looked different. He was not a particularly healthy person, from my memory, and he was beaming health. He said he had taken up yoga, was practicing meditation, and had become a vegetarian. I immediately started practicing all of those things.

During the summer, I had two courses—calculus and sociology. I had absolutely no interest in either of those subjects, or in most of the subjects I studied in college. So I spent the whole summer semester practicing *asanas*. Someone gave me a yoga book, and I started imitating all the postures. I somehow instinctively knew how to practice concentration, and I started to practice focusing all my attention on a piece of fruit or a flower. Overnight my ability to focus changed. I began to feel healthy. I did very little studying during that semester, but to my amazement, got A's in both of my subjects. From that point on, I had a pretty serious yoga practice, which I continued every day through my remaining two years of college.

After graduating from college, I decided to do what was most appealing to me—backpacking with a girlfriend in the Rockies. I spent a whole summer hiking and writing haiku poetry. It was a spiritual awakening for me. I read Thoreau's *Walden*. The combination of being in nature while reading about Thoreau's year living in the woods inspired me to spend a year living alone in a cabin on Cape Cod. That was really the turning point in my life.

When I first set out to do it, I had some qualms about being all alone. I had some friends helping me insulate the cabin. My last friend left on a dreary, rainy evening in mid-November. I said goodbye to him, and I felt this sinking feeling. As I walked back to the cabin, I found myself saying, "I am not alone." It immediately put my fears at rest, and I had an incredibly beautiful experience. There were times when friends came down. There were times when I would be with my family. But I spent the greater part of the year living alone and really taking a look at what I wanted to do with my life. I felt all of the social pressures such as, "You should get such and such a job, you should make so much money, you should be an accomplished whatever," dissolve.

Did you have parental support on this yearlong endeavor?

I didn't have family discouragement. I'm not sure I could call it support, but there wasn't opposition. My parents stepped back and allowed me to find out what I wanted to do. I felt free to choose my own life.

At some point, did a light bulb come on and you have a revelation of what to do with your life?

No. It happened naturally. There was one point when I got really restless. I admired my grandfather who was a very fine painter. I had studied art in college and thought that was a possibility. Around January, I picked up some paints, took out some paper, and began to do a watercolor. I was amazed at what came out. It was a very powerful experience. I began to get into drawing and painting, believing that I had found something. After a couple of months of doing this, all the aliveness had gone out of my drawing and my painting. There was no inspiration whatsoever. Then it just struck me—I am not interested in trying to create an identity for myself that is not me. I felt a new strength. There was a conviction that made me feel more centered. I got very clear about what I wanted to do—dedicate my life to yoga.

Fall was coming again. I had done the year in the woods. There was not that much appeal to do another. A yoga teacher from India was in the New York City area. One of my friends on the Cape had met him. She called me and said, "You've got to come down and meet this guy." I felt an irresistible pull. It was the strongest force I had ever felt.

I decided to take a trip and include New York City in it. I went up to New Hampshire to visit some friends, and the moment I got there, I felt I had to leave. I had to get to New York. I talked a friend into driving down, and we stopped in Westchester at his house and spent the night. He asked me to stick around the next day to spend some time with his family. I said, "Okay, but you might find me gone in the morning."

I woke up at four in the morning, took a subway into New York, a bus up to Monroe, and found out where the center was. I walked three or four miles with a backpack into these beautiful grounds and saw at a distance a group of people sitting on the lawn. As I got closer, I saw this little man with very dark skin, dressed in orange, with a pointer in his hand, chanting. I found out later that he was chanting Sanskrit grammar. I immediately began to connect with the Sanskrit. I understood it. It made sense to me, and I could pick it up very easily. I spent the next three years doing nothing but learning Sanskrit.

Was this an ashram *setting?*

It was an *ashram*, but shortly after that he ended up going to San Francisco to teach at the California Institute of Asian Studies. I asked him if I could study with him, and he said he was very happy to have me come along. He found a place where a group of people could live together and study Sanskrit intensively. That was what we did seven days a week. We would start at eight in the morning with a little bit of meditation, and then go until one-thirty eating a handful of sunflower seeds and a cup of tea midway through the morning. We would have the only meal of the day around one-thirty, picking up again at six in the evening and going until ten-thirty or eleven. We were getting between six and eight hours of Sanskrit every day, seven days a week, week in, week out, month in, month out. It continued that way for about two-and-a-half years.

What was your motivation?

His voice was extraordinary. Many levels of overtone and vibration were occurring so richly that I found it an incredible enjoyment to listen to him and then to duplicate him. Within the first week, I connected with the Sanskrit language. It was a spiritual homecoming. It was what I had always been looking for. It felt so nourishing to me on every level. Everything was new and fresh, and

I was so excited about the Sanskrit that I was learning. We chanted everything—the alphabet, nouns, verbs. We chanted *sutras* and Sanskrit literature. I could not get enough of this language. Sanskrit connected me to life.

Were you practicing asana *during this time?*

I had my own *asana* practice, and I continued to teach yoga. Sanskrit requires yoga. The form of yoga I teach incorporates sound, primarily to help people open up their resonating capacities. Yoga that includes sound is very helpful in learning Sanskrit. It's very difficult to learn Sanskrit without the application of yoga. It's a joy to learn it with yoga.

How were you able to access such a difficult language so easily?

I had never been a scholarly person or someone who was brilliant with languages. That was not the case at all. The thing that made Sanskrit so available to me was that it was the first thing I could put my whole heart, soul, and voice into. That was the key. Sanskrit has always been thought of as being a very difficult subject and language for Westerners to access. But I had a remarkable teacher who never tired of chanting the alphabet and the simplest grammatical forms over and over again.

I had a good voice, but yoga opened up my body to feel resonance. There was a way that I could follow my teacher and not hold myself back at all. So when he chanted, I would not hesitate to let my full voice come out. Through that process, Sanskrit became absolutely crystal clear to me. I saw how the language worked. Within a fairly short period of time, I found myself translating verses from various Sanskrit texts. Within nine months, the literature opened up to me, and I could understand it.

Why did you leave San Francisco?

I took a trip around the world with my teacher and eventually went to India. That was an incredible experience. It wasn't everything that I thought it was going to be. I thought traveling with the person whom I regarded as a great spiritual master and an extraordinary being would be the ultimate experience of my life. I had to come to terms with the fact that he was a human being who had defects and flaws. I went through a period of disillusionment. I was very angry that this human being was not perfect. It was a tough trip. It wasn't the heavenly journey that I had imagined. By the time we got to India, we had been through a lot on an emotional level. I reached the point where I felt my love for him and my connection to him as a human being. For me, that was a profound turning point, because it was also the place where I accepted my own self, not as a disciple who was less than him, but as spiritual friend and an equal. I matured a great deal.

India was a profound experience. I stayed there for three months. I went to south India with a friend and contracted hepatitis. I was so sick that I began to worry about whether I was going to make it back to the United States and see my family and friends again. I realized that the fear was draining my last bit of energy. I had to resign myself to the fact that I might not make it back. Then I let go. As soon as I let go, I began have a very spiritual experience of healing.

Fortunately, a very loving Muslim family who were friends of a friend took care of me. They were very kind and nursed me back to health. The mother of this family brought me fresh, hand-squeezed grape juice every couple of hours and that kept me going for a week until I could begin to eat solid foods again. My close friend, who had invited me, would pedal across Bangalore every morning at six and bring me the only herb that is known to cure hepatitis. It had to be ground up, mixed with milk, and taken early in the morning.

People have learned a lot more about what they have to do to stay healthy in India. I was not paying that much attention. I was very strong and in good shape when I went, but I wasn't vigilant with what I drank and ate. I was so absorbed in the experience of India that I actually learned how to ignore my body. At that point in my life I was young and feeling invincible. India proved to me that I wasn't invincible at all. I went four years later, in 1974, and I had a recurrence of hepatitis. Now I don't travel to India.

The Kumbha Mela was in 1974. Did you attend?

The Kumbha Mela had just ended as we arrived in Hardiwar, but there was still very much the feeling of it. It was a shock to me to see naked *sadhus* holding tridents walking down the middle of the street with dreadlocks down to their feet. I was going through a pretty profound cultural shock.

Where did your journey lead when you returned to the states?

It took me a good year or two before I really got my strength back. I became director at an *ashram* in New York, got married, and had a beautiful daughter named Brahmani. I continued with my Sanskrit studies. My teacher encouraged me to go back to college and get a degree in Sanskrit, so I went to Columbia University for a couple of years. It was good for me. I had spent too much time living strictly in a spiritual community. I was feeling a need to reconnect with the world. My experience in spiritual communities gave me a tendency to become isolated and feel different from the rest of the world, and I didn't like it. It wasn't comfortable. My years at Columbia were the beginning of a reintegration process for me.

Much of the study I had done up to that point had been based

on the chanting of Sanskrit, and enjoying the flow and the resonance. At Columbia, there was none of that. There was no emphasis on the proper pronunciation. But it was an opportunity to read
some great Sanskrit literature. Barbara Stoler Miller, a professor and
my advisor, loved to hear me chant, but most of the classes I took
were basically reading.

The most important part of my Columbia University experience was writing my master's thesis. I took a year to devote myself
to the *Yoga Sutras* of Patanjali. This was the next major, maybe *the*
major turning point in my life. I was beginning to take a deeper
look at the *Yoga Sutras*, and I came upon Georg Feuerstein's translation. He had done a great deal of research, and from his perspective,
it was time to go back to the original work and not be so dependent
on the commentaries. The whole commentarial tradition had basically been derived from a single source, which was Vyasa's original
commentary. Only a couple of twentieth century scholars had really
begun to challenge his commentary.

I began to accept that Vyasa's work was strong in some ways, but
weak in others. I read his commentary, and I began to do exactly
what Feuerstein was suggesting—take a deeper look at the *Yoga
Sutras*. It made sense to me to memorize the *sutras*. I found that after
memorizing them and having read a lot of the commentarial literature, the *sutras* began to gel inside me. I began to see interconnec-
tions and interrelationships between the *sutras* that, for me, were
much more meaningful than any commentary I had read. There was
so much more dimension and depth in the *sutras* internalized, than
there was in reading what somebody else had to say about them.
Intellectual tangents were not relevant to me. They may have been
relevant to the authors, but they were not relevant to my inner experience. It was the beginning of spiritual independence. It was time for
me to move out of the *ashram* environment and begin to do my own
work and my own teaching. Everything began to unfold.

Why had the time come to leave the ashram setting?

There were many reasons I felt the need to leave the *ashram*, but one of the biggest was to provide a home that was not in an isolated community for my daughter. It may have been a nice place for her as a small child, but she began to feel a sense of difference, some shame, and separation from other kids. Also, when I lived in a yoga community, my perspective became much too narrow.

You have one of the most resonant voices that I have ever heard. Is that a gift that you brought to Sanskrit or has Sanskrit given you that gift?

I have always had a good voice, but the chanting of Sanskrit and the practice of yoga has deepened that. One of the beautiful things about Sanskrit is that the resonance keeps opening up over the years. The clarity of the pronunciation is equivalent to clarity of mind. More resonance is the expanding of energy. The focus on the five mouth positions, the pinpointed focus of your tongue and your lips, which is something that the Sanskrit language naturally draws your attention to, continues to get clearer.

Sanskrit opens up a state of meditation or *sattva*, a state of crystal clarity and light. You make the conversion from identifying with the body as being a solid block, separate from everything else, to being this fluid, supple energy field that senses and feels everything around it. We are going to recognize, and it seems to be happening now, that Sanskrit is as essential a tool to the process of yoga as *asana* is. Since America is physical and athletic culture, our tendency has been to gravitate towards practicing the postures, and that was the first thing that I went for. I love that aspect of yoga and I still practice it, but I don't give it any more importance than the power of sound and the power of language. Sanskrit is a highly specialized, technical language designed to direct this body, mind, and energy field complex to its ultimate fulfillment.

Vyaas Houston is the founder and director of the American Sanskrit Institute. He studied Sanskrit with Dr. Ramamurti S. Mishra and at Columbia University where he earned a Master of Arts degree. After teaching Sanskrit and yoga for more than fifteen years, he discovered in 1987 a successful method for teaching Sanskrit based on the yoga model of Patanjalis' *Yoga Sutras*. His Sanskrit training course has provided thousands of people with the opportunity to discover their own unique relationship with Sanskrit. He is the author of *Sanskrit by Cassette* and has recorded and translated many Sanskrit classics.

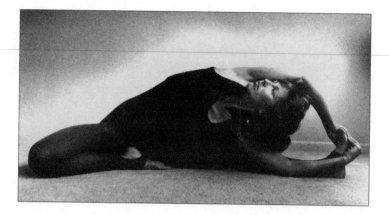

SANDRA SUMMERFIELD KOZAK

PHOENIX

How did you become a yoga teacher?

My first yoga teacher, who liked to call himself Crazy Bob, taught a yoga class that consisted of four asanas—cobra, forward bend, twist and *savasana*. To this day he likes to say that while he didn't know a lot about yoga, he was really good at making yoga teachers. This was 1971 and the understanding of yoga, then often called yogurt, was very limited. Crazy Bob was the only teacher in Reno at that time.

One day, after I had gone to about three of his classes, he called and said that he had a problem and asked me to substitute teach his next class for him. I said, "I don't know anything about yoga." But he pleaded, "Someone has to be there and you can do the poses. So just go in and do the poses and let them follow you." He wouldn't take "no" for an answer, so I finally agreed.

Over the next couple of years, he kept repeating this same behavior, but each time it was for more and more classes. First, it was one class, then three, and so on until finally one day he said, "I have to go to New York and will be gone for three months. Please take over all my classes for me." (I had been studying on my own by this time, so I knew more than four poses.) After more unrelenting persuasion, I finally agreed.

It took only a few days of Bob's four classes per week teaching schedule for me to realize two things—yoga was improving my health and life, and I didn't know what I was doing. I had been studying books like crazy, but that wasn't enough. So I began going to weekend trainings in Grass Valley and Sacramento, but the more I learned the more I knew that I didn't know anything. Then I was given the wonderful opportunity to move to San Francisco and attend the Institute for Yoga Teacher Education (now called the Iyengar Institute). Immersed in the Institute's training, I was in heaven learning psychology, philosophy, anatomy, physiology, meditation, *asana*, and teaching procedures. I was walking, talking, eating, and dreaming yoga.

In 1975, Mr. Iyengar came to San Francisco and gave a five-day seminar. I was so lucky to be allowed to attend. Mr. Iyengar was amazing, and I learned an incredible amount in those few days. I knew I had found my teacher. I began going to his three-week intensive trainings in India.

When I moved back to Reno, I began teaching yoga full-time. I designed and taught a yoga program for the University of Nevada-Reno and the Truckie Meadows Community College. I continued to go back to San Francisco for more study. To be able to continue to learn, I had to drive five hours each way to those workshops in San Francisco, as well as make arrangements for my children and housing for myself. It was expensive and difficult, but there was never a question about doing it.

Are you still a part of the Iyengar tradition?

I spent fourteen years studying with Mr. Iyengar and his senior teachers. When the certification program began Mr. Iyengar gave us our certifications. There were only three levels at that time, so there was a long time of study and practice between levels. While I continued to study, I didn't elect to be politically involved in that way.

The last time I was in India with Mr. Iyengar, I suffered a very serious injury. It was no one's fault, just an unfortunate circumstance that changed my ability to do *asanas* and the way I had to practice. The injury took three years to heal and the scar tissue that formed created permanent changes in my body.

During those three years of healing, I became interested in studying Patanjali's *Yoga Sutras*. I was again blessed with more fabulous teachers. And that's when I first came to understand that *asana* is only a small part of yoga, not the whole subject.

What aspects of yoga played a part in your recovery?

The injury was very unusual and very severe. The origin of the biceps femoris (one of the hamstring muscles) was almost torn away from its attachment to the sitting bone, and the sciatic nerve was badly pulled. Almost any stretching or strengthening move I did reinjured it. I learned a great deal through this injury and its healing process. Now I say to students, "Find the teacher who has had to work with their own injuries, and you will find a teacher that has a lot of information about that part of the body." Mr. Iyengar taught us this self-investigation style of learning. I used his teachings then, during the healing process, and I continue to use his teachings every day. The injury became a way to evolve, learn, and grow.

So asana *was the big key?*

The *injury* was the big key. Each time I would try to study or practice any forward or backward movement, more pain and injury was created. With that happening over and over again, I learned a great respect for the injury as a teacher, that I couldn't take anything for granted, and that I had to honor and take from my body only what it wanted to give me. I became more interested in the breath as the vehicle to my practice of *asana*. It taught me what Joel Kramer calls "playing the edge." Joel teaches that you go to the point of stretch that you can maintain and then you wait there until the body releases and relaxes. You accept the stretch and move to the new "edge" and wait again. This "playing the edge" style became my practice. I began to work with my body at a much deeper level than I was able to before. I also started studying *pranayama* and meditation.

I was not only dealing with the body, but I was also dealing with the whole psychology of yoga. The word *asana* can be split into three roots: *as*, which in Sanskrit means "to be" or "to breathe"; *san*, which in Sanskrit means "to bring together"; and *na*, which in Sanskrit means "that which is eternal." So the word *asana* can be translated to mean "pose" or "posture," or it can be interpreted from its three roots to mean "to be or to breathe together with that which is eternal." This seems like a clearer statement of what yoga really is and that is the change that I made through the injury.

A lot of our lives and actions are ego-driven. When the completed pose is the goal and the ego is the driving force toward that goal, injury is very available. My injury allowed me to see this, see yoga, and see my practice in a new way. It was one of the best things that could have happened to me.

You have become very involved in the European yoga tradition. How did you start teaching in Europe and what are some observations you may have made, particularly with respect to the quality of teaching in both America and Europe?

I was invited to teach in the U.K. eight years ago for Lendrick Lodge in Callandar and for the Scottish Yoga Teachers Association's annual conference. Di Kendal, then president of the British Wheel of Yoga and Secretary General of the European Union of Yoga (EUY) was an honored guest at that conference. She liked my teaching and later recommended me to the EUY. They invited me to teach the next year in Switzerland for their annual conference. During the next three years of teaching the EUY conferences, I had the very good fortune to be invited to sit in on their board and pedagogical meetings. They were then deciding on the completed requirements for their Initial Teacher Training Program, which was later adopted and ratified by their eighteen member countries. Training standards had been discussed for about twenty years and had been intently worked on for the previous six years.

Also, over the course of my annual teaching in seven other European countries, I learned about teacher training programs and witnessed the teachers they produced. I would return to America and see certification programs that were one weekend, a week, two weeks, or a month.

The European Union's initial four-year, five-hundred hour training program is very well rounded and delivers information on all aspects of yoga. This initial training produces good teachers who work from a solid foundation. In Europe, they believe that it takes time to grow a teacher, time for them to develop as people and as responsible and knowledgeable teachers. The five-hundred hours could be accomplished in less than four years time, but the feeling there is that the evolutionary changes and development of the student into a teacher takes longer. If this development does not have time to take place, the student will be sharing—through their teaching—their unresolved issues.

The process of yoga is not just about movement of the body. Yoga is a practice of compressed evolution to clean up the different levels of consciousness by bringing those issues and experiences, which are no longer visible to us, forward to make them visible. Patanjali's *Yoga Sutras* tell us that those old experiences that are now a part of our unconscious mind give impulse and come forward, without our awareness, to create actions and thoughts. In yoga, we say that the invisible must become visible to be eradicated. Moving these old unconscious experiences that drive our actions out and letting go of them is the cleansing process within the practice of yoga—the evolutionary growth to becoming a human being and to a state of joy.

Is yoga an older tradition in Europe than in America?

Yes. I found a more mature attitude in the European students as a whole. I like to go back to Europe each year because of the level at which the students receive the teaching. And I love teaching European teachers. They are the best students. They receive at such a high level. In fact, we all learn together from the information they bring forward. It's lovely.

The general quality of teaching is better in Europe because the educational requirements are higher there. For example, in Finland, they require eight years of initial teacher training, and their yoga teachers are seen as health professionals, like doctors. I am hoping that our country adopts high standards of yoga training requirements so that we gain a high level of professionalism within the field of yoga.

The issue of certification standards should be answered by a series of questions. How do you want yoga portrayed in America? What do you want yoga to be able to accomplish in America? The answer to those questions will tell you at what level teachers need to be trained. The teacher training isn't the same training you get when you go to yoga class. It's also about learning how to teach yoga.

The EUY and International Yoga Studies, which has brought the European Union's initial four-year teacher training program into America, both require two years of yoga training before application can be made. That is two years of class time, not teacher training. International Yoga Studies gives credit for past yoga teacher training, but not past yoga class experience. We expect our students to continue to attend yoga classes while in our program, because that is a part of their evolutionary process.

What was your inspiration for creating International Yoga Studies?

After twenty-seven years of work in yoga, I have come to see it as a subject incredibly valuable to people's lives. It's not just the physical movements, which in America are often called yoga. Yoga is also a resource for so many issues that plague our planet today. Yoga works to create better self-esteem, to lessen or eliminate the effects of fear (which breeds defense, which creates offense, which ends ultimately in war), to create better health and a general sense of well-being, and to strengthen our ability to relate to others, our planet, and ourselves. The practice of yoga creates more comfort on all levels in people's lives. But yoga can only be that resource if taught by educated teachers who themselves understand what yoga is.

As our consciousness develops, we naturally move away from a polarized individual perspective, into the more "we"-oriented mind. We are in touch with the idea that "kind to you" equates to "kind to me." We not only learn to manage our own energy systems, but to contribute to the energy system of the collective whole—of humanity. As Buckminster Fuller told us, "At a certain stage of development, you do not select the work that you do based on your desires, but rather by seeing and filling the position that needs filling, and doing the job that needs to be done." By creating good teachers of an invaluable subject, International Yoga Studies ultimately contributes to the larger community and to the collective "we." By assisting in training teachers who are capable of working responsibly, clearly, and safely with their students, a space for the understanding and use of the many benefits of yoga is created.

As each consciousness in our country grows, we all grow. By serving the collective "we," we serve each other and ourselves. It is this service that has inspired International Yoga Studies.

Do European yoga teachers offer a more well-rounded practice to their students than American yoga teachers, whose practice may be firmly fixated on asana?

Yes. The Europeans tend to be much more focused on a general program than we are here. We're culturally biased and based here. And our culture tends to be more focused on the body. In yoga, there is much more movement to be made than just with the physical body. So I think the Europeans are generally more well-rounded in their teaching and their practice, although Americans have much more *asana* information.

I don't mean to say that everyone in America is fixated on *asana*. But many teachers who say that they are teaching hatha yoga are actually only teaching *asana*, sometimes with a little *pranayama* thrown in. *Asana*, hatha yoga, and *raja* yoga are not all the same thing. *Asana* is a small part of the practice of both hatha yoga and *raja* yoga. But there is so much more to yoga than *asana* practice.

Do you think the Christian heritage of America creates resistance to the philosophical and spiritual teachings of yoga?

Christianity, or any religion, is perfectly supported by yoga. Yoga is not a religion or a belief system—it is a practice. And through the practice of yoga, evolution of the person's consciousness results. I think the problem a fundamentalist thinker would have with a philosophical system like yoga would be they might think it is somehow tied to Hinduism or some other religious persuasion.

Actually, someone who is theistic or non-theistic can practice yoga. If there is no god in your reality, yoga is fantastic because it is a very practical way to develop your consciousness into a comfortable state of abiding happiness. Yoga does not define style, and supports any and all religious belief.

Man's oldest search has been for happiness. The philosophies that came out of what would later become India were to appease that search. The six Eastern philosophical systems were born from the approximate time of 2700 B.C. to 600 B.C. Each presents a view of reality that is designed to find a way to move from a state of unhappiness into a state of abiding happiness, which, they profess, should be the natural enlightened human condition.

Yoga is one of the six philosophical systems that came about during the time of the Samkhya culture. Samkhya was not a religion. It is a way of understanding reality, and yoga is the practice component of this way of understanding.

Yoga suggests you can relieve yourself of suffering by remaining focused and detached. In the first chapter, *Sadhana Pada*, of the *Yoga Sutras*, Patanjali tells us to continually remain focused and practice detachment. Being focused and detached will bring the abiding experience of happiness—your natural state of being. By releasing the past, you wake up and discover what already exists within you. Yoga is also about consciousness management and evolution. It's about being able to undo that which binds your consciousness, holds you down, and restricts you to the suffering experience.

Can one truly remove suffering?

Yes. First by understanding the nature of the suffering. Most people live going from riding high to feeling low with constant ups and downs throughout their lives. This type of living (we could call it the "soap opera" approach) is about being very happy and very unhappy, and it wastes a lot of energy. When this energy is continually focused on the present moment without attachment, there is much more energy available for the very intense moment-to-moment experience of joy. Yoga offers techniques for resolving the issues that create the ups and downs, the "soap opera," and for managing the previously wasted energy into a stronger experience of the present moment.

When I think of an example of detachment, I remember a time when I attended a Buddhist training with the Dalai Lama. Once, when he was speaking about his life, he suddenly started to cry. He didn't try to explain it or suppress it, even though he was lecturing to hundreds of people at the time. He cried for several minutes, and then dried his eyes, blew his nose, and went on with the lecture. Some part of his past had come to light. He allowed the experience, and then released it and let it go. Experiences that are painful when they first happen are also often experienced as painful when we let them go. In front of hundreds of people, the Dalai Lama experienced, let go, and then went on with his lecturing.

It isn't so much that the suffering doesn't exist. In life, painful events happen and there is pain. But, instead of experiencing them and letting them go, most of us attach and carry the pain from the past with us, on and on throughout our lives. You meet people that have had some experience that has crippled them. They can't move on, and their past experience determines their present moments, so that they are like a broken record replaying the same part over and over again. This is the antithesis of yoga. Detachment doesn't mean that I never attach to anything or anyone. Attachment is the nature of our ego energy and a necessary part of our consciousness. Patanjali didn't say, "Don't attach." He said, "Detach." Detachment is about being able to let go of what I have been attached to and move on.

This is tricky, because we use attachment in a variety of ways. Often we use attachment to create the illusion of security that then allows us to feel more comfortable. Life is a fearful event if you are attached to it. When we structure our lives by attaching ourselves to places, people, and things to do, we are able to avoid some of this fear that is inherent in life. Structure is very comforting. We like to structure everything—our time, our lives, our possessions, and our view of ourselves. We say, "I'm the kind of person who gains five pounds if I even look at a piece of cheesecake." We know that physiologically, that's not even possible. But we continue to define ourselves, wrapping these definitions around ourselves so we can know who we are. Structure provides us with a sense of security, but it also eliminates creativity.

Also, we like to attach meaning to everything that happens to us. It gives us a sense of security and eases our reactions to very difficult happenings. For instance, if we have had a loss and we are able to attach some meaning to that loss, it softens the experience and makes the pain somehow easier to bear. It's comforting to us to know that it wasn't "all for nothing."

But the universe and our lives are full of random events and there isn't always meaning to assign. When we constantly insist on assigning meaning to everything, we separate ourselves from the full experience of our lives, we interfere with our experience of true faith, and we eliminate the Unknowable.

I ask students to see all life in front of them and to remember that death is behind them, and to remain aware of this whole perspective at all times. This simple idea heightens the awareness of *now*. There's no time for denial or drifting, no time for depression. There is just *now*. When you are awake and conscious, it isn't a matter of "going with the flow" or the "path of least resistance." Being awake or enlightened is living on the razor's edge. If you are comfortable, it usually means you are sleeping in one form or another. The razor's edge is where the awareness is, where *now* is.

What does your personal practice consist of?

I try to make my whole life my yoga. There is my regular *asana, pranayama,* and meditation practice. But I focus on the rest of my life as an even larger part of my yoga practice. Yoga is about the evolution of consciousness. It's about the continual knowing and letting go of that which creates Sandra working from any one reactive place. My focus is to remain awake and work from a position of "causing" my life, rather than being "effected" by it.

The attitudes I find in my poses reflect the attitudes I have and use in the rest of my life. I think of Patanjali's *Yoga Sutras* as a mirror to see ourselves in this way and as a map. The practices and techniques of yoga are a variety of ways to see yourself. The goal seeking, the irritation, the loving, the passivity, or whatever you find in the pose, you will find other places in your life—in your relationships, in your professional life.

Yoga also gives us a map for our evolutionary journey into Union, *Samadhi*, Being. It is the process of seeing what is making us uncomfortable and practicing techniques designed for evolving into a more comfortable, joyful, and whole consciousness.

Sandra Summerfield Kozak has studied and taught yoga for twenty-seven years. She was Iyengar-certified in 1976, and has studied with many world-renowned yogis, including Swami Muktananda, Baba HariDass, and T.K.V. Desikachar. She holds a Masters of Science degree with her final thesis on "The Physiological Effect of Yoga: Asana, Pranayama, Meditation." Sandra is the founder and director of International Yoga Studies, an educational organization dedicated to creating a standardized certification program that supports quality education for yoga teachers in North America. Additionally, she is the Vice President of Unity in Yoga and the Secretary General of the World Yoga Union. Sandra teaches annually in Europe and monthly throughout North America.

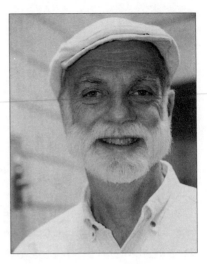

MARTIN PIERCE
ATLANTA

How long have you been following the path of yoga?

I started in 1968. I was teaching political science at New York University. I was involved in the peace movement, and the civil rights movement, and I was teaching a lot of courses. So I was under a lot of stress. Somebody suggested I try yoga as a way of dealing with it. There were only a few places teaching yoga in New York City at that time. Eventually, I decided that I was more interested in the yoga than in political science.

In 1970, I went on a spiritual search. I had a small inheritance that enabled me to quit my job and to travel. I didn't have a lot of money, so I traveled overland to India. I flew to Luxembourg and then took all kinds of conveyances. I hitchhiked in a coal truck across Turkey.

Did you ride a camel?

I got on a camel, but I wouldn't say I accomplished any part of the journey on a camel. I rode in all kinds of little cars and buses and trucks all the way across to India. I spent some time traveling around India looking for a teacher. I went down into Sri Lanka checking out Buddhist teachers. There were lots of people who were available to teach yoga, but they were teaching the same thing that I had learned in America, or they were charlatans. I didn't find anybody that first trip that I really felt good about.

In 1972, I went back to India and looked for a teacher in a more determined way. The first time I had been doing some sight-seeing and staying at different *ashrams*. I met a man who I really respected that I had met on my first trip to India. He advised me that there were two really fine yoga teachers in India. He said one was fierce—it was Iyengar, of course—and the other he said was gentle. I had had a back problem for some years. At that time, it caused me to stoop over. The yoga that I had done before had not helped my back. In fact, at times it irritated my condition and made it worse. I decided I had better go see the gentle teacher.

You were practicing yoga and your back was still hurting. What kept you going?

There was peace. There was something about the people who did yoga. A certain spiritual atmosphere kept drawing me back.

Please continue.

I went to see Desikachar in Madras. I had already been through Madras three times in my travels. I went back on the hard boards of third class railway carriages and met Desikachar. He did not especially impress me at first, because he seemed ordinary, so unassuming. The teachers that I had met before dressed the part, wearing gorgeous robes with disciples around them. They lived in *ashrams*. He was just living with his family and teaching out of his own home. There was this old guy sitting on the porch reading the paper. I had no idea that the old guy was the great Krishnamacharya—B.K.S. Iyengar's teacher, K. Pattabhi Jois' teacher, Indra Devi's teacher. Desikachar looked like some middle-class guy, but I had come all the way to Madras to meet him.

Desikachar said, "If you're interested in studying with me, come back next week." I hung around Madras for a week, and the next week I showed up. He said, "Oh, you're still here. Come back next week and I'll give you a lesson." This was very different from the treatment I received from all the other teachers around India who were eager for me to be a student. They thought it would be great to have an American study with them. But Desikachar was different. As his father, Krishnamacharya, would have done, he was seeing if I was serious. He was testing me out by making me wait a couple of weeks. (Desikachar tells a story about how when he asked his father to study; Krishnamacharya made him come at three in the morning for lessons, when Desikachar was working a regular nine-to-five job). I thought, "Well, I've come all this way. I might as well take some lessons." So I stuck around.

The next week I met with Desikachar. I did the exercises and breathing he showed me. They were different from what I had done before. They were not the classical poses that I had been taught. But I noticed that my back was getting better, and also, I was feeling calmer. Something was happening at some other level than just the physical.

Desikachar had said to me that he would not teach me unless I agreed to stay for three months. I said, "Okay." But in my mind I was saying, "I'll give him a month and we'll see." I lived at the Theosophical Society where I had a little room. India in those days was extremely cheap. You could live well for a hundred dollars a month, so the money lasted for a long time. I wound up staying a year. Towards the end of that year Desikachar trained me to be a yoga teacher.

I came to Atlanta, which happened to be where my ex-wife was with my son, and started looking for a job. I thought, "While I'm looking for a job, I might as well teach yoga." This was the ideal time for that to happen, because in 1973 there was a big upsurge and interest in yoga. People starting coming, and pretty soon I didn't have time to look for a real job anymore.

Margaret, my wife, was one of my first students. These days it's very clear that you are not supposed to date your students, and I think that's a good principle, but I did date her. The following year she and I went to India together. In March 1975, we were married in India with Desikachar as a witness. We came back and started The Pierce Program.

We have continued to study with Desikachar. We have invited him here a couple of times, and we have studied with him in Europe and India. It seems that there is always more to learn. Every time I see him I think, "Now I understand yoga," but he always has more to teach. At first it was mostly on a physical level, though we did study the *Yoga Sutras*. As time has gone on, it's become more and more spiritual. The content of what I teach has become more spiritual.

In what ways?

If you teach the *asanas* and *pranayama* in the proper way, it's going to be spiritual. In our tradition, the definition of *asana* is a posture in which you are strong and stable, comfortable and relaxed, and intelligently aware of what you are doing. If you do that, something happens in your body. You slow down and focus. You become aware of deeper reality. When students ask for it, we do chanting with the *asanas*. We do visualizations with the *asanas*. I either talk about the yoga philosophy at the end of class, or I read stories that have some kind of spiritual background.

It sounds as though you are as much a minister as a yoga teacher.

My father teases me about that. He refers to my students as my parishioners. I would not call myself a minister, but these days people are increasingly coming to yoga for something spiritual.

What I am not able to do, and what I wish I could do, is keep an ongoing relationship with all the people who come to yoga class to help them with their spiritual journey. Someday, I hope I will get to the point where I can do that. At present, somebody will come to an eight-week meditation class, but when the course ends, they are on their own. They need some way of formally continuing their spiritual journey.

The best way to teach is by example. Desikachar is a very spiritual person. He is a very loving, caring, gentle person. He is serious, but he has a wonderful sense of humor. When he teaches, he conveys that. Not just by his words, but by his presence. Yoga is about *ahimsa*, caring. The *Yoga Sutras* say that. If you do yoga in a good way then you are more caring, first of all towards yourself, and then towards your friends, your family, and society.

What led you into political science and political activism?

My family was very political, but very conservative. Politics was always discussed in my house. I knew people who were active in politics. It was natural for me to act politically. It was something I understood. Organizing political groups came very easy to me. The thing that was hard for me to say was, "I need to change myself." That's the most important thing before I try to change other people.

My roots go back to the Episcopalian church, where service was important. I had a very influential grandmother who was active in our church. She was an example of a person who helps others. At first, I thought politics was the way to change the world.

In the sixties, there was so much strife and conflict, and it was upsetting to me. For instance, the conflict among the people on my side in the peace movement. I was in a peace march in Maryland, and there was a Marine guard outside a base. A couple of the people I was marching with went up to this Marine guard and started screaming at him and telling him what a terrible person he was to be in the Marines. He was standing there very calmly, talking to them in a reasonable way. And I thought, "Who's for peace? The people who are screaming or this Marine?"

I thought what may be most important is a fundamental change in myself and in people, prior to being able to change the world and making it more peaceful. People have got to be ready to be peaceful. I think that idea was fermenting in me all the time. Again and again, I would try to convince people by rational argument that a certain way was the way to go. Argument is not a very effective way of changing people for the better. Logic is not very effective. You need to work at a deeper level, and yoga touches that deeper level. Yoga helps people to be more truly caring towards others.

You can try to manipulate people, coerce them, pay them, or persuade them rationally. But the most powerful way is to help people become more peaceful inside themselves. If I get down to who I really am, I am not an angry person. I don't think anybody is an angry person when we get down to who they most deeply are. And discovering that spiritual core is what yoga is about.

Do you still consider yourself an active member of the peace movement?

I am not active, but I am concerned and may at some time return to it.

The people that I always liked to be with were the Quakers. I was a Quaker and I attended Quaker meetings. Often we would just stand silently with a sign and try to be caring towards those who favored military action.

You have been periodically traveling to India for close to thirty years. What has been your perception of the yoga movement in India over that time?

When I first went in 1970, yoga was not at all respected in India. People who did yoga were considered old-fashioned. Indians were interested in becoming modern, in Westernizing, in earning money. Yoga has become much more popular in India, because they have seen that people in the West do yoga. Because of the West, they now appreciate their own heritage more.

Have you ever been sick traveling to India?

Very sick. Many times! When I would come back to Atlanta, the people at DeKalb General Hospital laboratories would say, "We're so glad to see you again. You brought us something interesting to look at." Now I am extremely careful, and I have been quite lucky the last few years. I stay in one apartment where there is a cook whom I trust, and I eat out as little as possible. The last time I got sick there I was in a four-star hotel. Also, I keep myself in better shape that I used to. When I first went to India, I traveled over land.

I was pretty exhausted and my resistance was not good. When I went into little towns, I had to starve or eat what they gave me. Now I do my yoga practice, so my resistance to infection is better, I think.

What does your practice consist of?

I always do yoga early in the morning, first thing when I get up. I do forty minutes of *asanas*, five or ten minutes of breathing, and ten minutes of meditation and visualizations. I also do a few stretches at different times during the day and at night before I go to sleep.

Is visualization different from meditation?

It is and it isn't. Meditation involves finding an object that has some characteristics that take you toward your deepest, most spiritual Self. It can be done different ways. If somebody wants to have the feeling of serenity and strength, they might look at a snow-capped mountain outside and that will help them move in the direction. If a person needs to be calm, they might look at a pool of water and meditate on that. Or maybe a certain *mantra* will help them. Desikachar gave me certain personal *mantras* and concepts to focus on. That's like a doctor giving a prescription.

Tomorrow I've got a very busy travel schedule. If I visualize myself doing that tonight before I go, then I think I'll be happy about it when I do it. I'll be appreciating the moment, and I'll also be less likely to make stupid mistakes, like forgetting the car keys or making a wrong turn on the highway. I won't be perfect, but I'm convinced I'll travel better. That's an ordinary everyday visualization to help me get through tomorrow.

What is your definition of success?

When you say success, you have to talk about the opposite side of the coin, which is failure. You are introducing a dualism. I just try to think about doing a good job, helping people, and being grateful. In our society, you can't help but think about success, because the media constantly emphasizes it. We are urged to be successful, and the emphasis on that is really distracting to a lot of people.

At the end of the day, I may look back and say, "I had a lot of good moments today," but I won't score it. I won't say, "This was a successful day." I'll just be grateful for good things that happened.

I don't like to put negative ideas in my mind, because it sets up a struggle. I might say, "I need to be more giving." I find it very helpful to think every day, "What am I grateful for?" A good relationship with my daughters. That I am in this wonderful studio, and there are bamboo plants outside the window.

I used to have a tendency to think about all the things that go wrong. But when I can think about what I am grateful for, I realize there is an enormous amount of things that are wonderful in my life.

Martin Pierce has practiced yoga since 1968 and has been a student of T.K.V. Desikachar since 1972. With his wife, Margaret, he founded The Pierce Program and co-authored *Yoga for Your Life: A Practice Manual of Breath and Movement*. He has written for *Yoga Journal*, *Yoga International*, *Viniyoga*, and other publications. He is the former president of Viniyoga America. Martin received a B.A. from Yale and an M.A. in American History from the University of Wisconsin, and taught Political Science at New York University. Martin was active in the Peace and Civil Rights Movements from 1957 to 1969. The father of three regularly attends and occasionally teaches at his Episcopal Church.

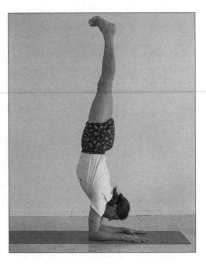

GABRIEL HALPERN
CHICAGO

Please describe your teaching style.

I am not one of those teachers who just sticks to postures. I feel you teach yoga, you don't teach *asanas*.

I hurt my back in high school and was misdiagnosed. I have a condition called spondylolisthesis which is where the vertebrae breaks off from the pedicle of the vertebral body. It can't be surgically repaired, or if it can, they didn't have the technology at that time. The osteopath who saw me was not a very astute practitioner, because he simply gave me a back brace. I had gone to his office in the shape of a scythe, and after six weeks, I still couldn't even bend down to bring my fingers level to my knees. I somehow managed to gut my way through playing high school football, which only made my condition worse.

I didn't understand the wounded healer myth at the time, but it certainly was in the background propelling me to find surcease from my constant low-grade irritation that was my traveling companion, and still is. By wounded healer, I mean you seek your own path while trying to find help for yourself, and then as a result of what you learn, you pass it on. Very few people who are healers in the healing arts have not come through a transformational experience themselves, and usually it's because they were hurt badly in some way.

Because I am a wounded healer, I can appeal to people. When you show your students that you are limited and you are injured, rather than losing respect for you, they see your humanity. Because you are more like your students, your relationship is closer. The other model is idolizing teachers, putting them upon a pedestal, feeling they are very beyond you, and hoping to aspire to their level.

I have often wondered if I had not gotten in that fight and hurt my back, would I have discovered yoga and gone around the world to meet the people I have met? If I could rewrite it now, so that I would not have this pain but not be assured that my life would end up the way it has so far, would I do it? No. I would rather have the pain and accept the way my life has been, because beautiful things have happened. That's finding the blessing behind the curse. It's not just a matter of re-framing it. There are so many different teachings about adversity bringing something forth from it. There is no resurrection without a crucifixion. There is wisdom to be garnered in every life experience.

You became a householder later in life.

I married at forty-three and had my first child at forty-four.

How has becoming a husband and father impacted your yoga practice and other aspects of your life?

I came to the stage in my life where I was ready for what the truth of relationship had to offer. Since I wanted a family, I don't have regrets. When you are ready, it becomes your path. It doesn't take you away from your path. Yoga is a lifestyle. If you are really doing yoga, your life is seamless with your yoga.

Does relationship mean that my practice has to suffer? If I am still holding on to my old image of practicing as much as when I was single, then yes, I could say my practice suffers. Because I have an injury, I have to spend some time just to make my back feel good. It may not be as many hours as it used to be. Sometimes it might be only maintenance, but that's okay. I have accepted the fact that I don't practice as much, but the practices are not just ends to themselves. They serve a purpose—to develop your consciousness, to help bring presence of mind into whatever you are doing.

I have seen many other yogis whose hatha yoga practice looks like Cirque de Soleil—very advanced and beautiful. But the amount of time they spend autistically rocking to the sound of their own *Om*, at the expense of the ability to be intimate with another human being, is not a trade-off I want to make. You can become very imbalanced by one-sidedly doing your practice. We are not supposed to cultivate the spirit at the expense of a body, nor are we supposed to be hedonistically involved in the body without acknowledging the truth of the spirit. I don't think you are supposed to be alone all the time, or totally merged with another human being, so you can't bear being without them. It's about balance.

As a teacher, it is so important to have somebody who sees you behind the scenes. I married an Irish woman who puts me in my place the way nobody else can, even more than Mr. Iyengar. Mr. Iyengar stops once you are outside of the class! But as for my wife, all I hear, God bless her soul, is "Oh, Master of Awareness, time to take out the garbage!"

When I was younger, I had a monastic and celibate *ashram* experience. I have had so many years of being by myself, and devoting hours and hours to practice and cloistered situations. If you are going to be involved with relationship, then you certainly still need some time for yourself. I appreciate those situations, but I don't need them desperately, as if I can't function without them. I can find centering in other ways. The fire doesn't matter—whether it's monastic fire or the fire of relationships. Relationship is a crucible. It refines you, puts you through changes, and purifies you.

My relationship with my kids became a new aspect of yoga. It's *bhakti* yoga and *karma* yoga. Devotion and right action. It's an opportunity to merge the knowledge that I have from the books into the practical aspect of my daily life. I am not resentful of the entry of these people into my life as if somehow they are preventing me from following my path. They help me to fulfill my path and further my path.

How did you discover yoga?

I first experienced yoga as an acting major at Queens College in the sixties. The drama department taught a whole series of tai chi exercises, Chinese acrobatics, and yoga stretches, but they didn't tell you that was what they were teaching.

Two years later, I moved to Kentfield, California. I happened to live right across the street from the College of Marin. I was summa cum hippie at the time. As I was walking across the campus, I noticed a *kundalini* yoga course was being offered. People were doing a powerful breath of fire exercise where you rapidly inhale and exhale. It looked really dynamic and captured my attention, so I took a class. I was looking for transition out of psychedelics. Something really appealed to me about the natural high you could get from working your breath that way, probably because I was still hooked on the feelings of psychedelics. I stayed with the *kundalini* yoga people for six years doing my practice.

Kundalini yoga is very powerful and you develop a lot of concentration, strength of mind. The meditations are focused on *mantra* and the hatha yoga is geared towards holding positions. It is very esoteric in terms of integrating the *chakras*. It didn't offer me much in terms of alignment details and actual healing at a structural level. It gave me some flexibility, but it didn't really teach me the therapeutic knowledge that would take me further along my journey.

In 1976, I moved to Miami and saw a yoga advertisement featuring a very athletic hard body. I went to a class and it turned out to be my introduction into Iyengar yoga. The teacher, Bobbie Goldin who was a pint-sized practitioner, was doing fantastic arm balances and backbends. I knew I had made a quantum leap by just walking into her class.

I am still an Iyengar practitioner, but I openly admit that I am an opportunist. If I found anything else that was the next step, I would turn my attention to that. But I have never seen another yoga that has the depth of refinement and profundity. I have never found another yogi whose life experience has been as evolved as Mr. Iyengar's. I studied Iyengar yoga for eleven years before I actually went to India. I went in 1987 and 1989 for teacher intensives and in 1996 for general classes. What impressed me most about Iyengar yoga was that each teacher I studied with was teaching a system. They were all very unique and individual, and yet each one sang the praises of the master that had influenced them.

What led you to Chicago?

In 1984, I had finished a masters program and was in a holding pattern. I had taken a couple of six-week training courses at the San Francisco Institute of Yoga. I intended to finish my Iyengar training, and then take an East/West Ph.D. course at the California Institute of Integral Studies. In the interim, I came to Chicago to see my brother, which I had done over the years.

During this particular visit, a teacher at a local yoga center offered me a job. Chicago would not have been on my list of twenty cities I wanted to move to, but I was thousands of dollars in the hole from my student loans. This uncanny counter-intuitive voice said, "There is really something right about coming to a freezing cold environment after having been known as 'the tan yogi.'" (I earned this moniker, not only because I had a bitching tan, but also I wore a lot of tone-on-tone tan to match the tone of my skin.)

Iyengar yoga was not being taught at the yoga center where I became the primary teacher. I brought in all the props that are in the style of Iyengar yoga, and the students slurped me up like a dry plant needing water. I had such a warm reception the first month I was in Chicago. The students took me around the city and made me feel so at home. I really felt a connection.

It's an amazing thing when you look at your journey. Sometimes you find where you are going by going somewhere else. Even though you think your will has been thwarted, you have really been guided, but you don't even know it. I have been doing my practice for twenty-seven years now, and I hope to be doing it for another twenty-seven years. As one rabbi said, "Turn aging into saging."

What influenced you to merge men's issues with yoga?

I was deeply affected by Robert Bly. *Iron John* was the first book that influenced me to look at my relationship with my father. He died when I was young, and we didn't really have a chance to heal. Later, I had an astral experience of him returning to me and giving me a certain blessing that it was okay for me to go on in my life. Wounds you experienced as a child can still affect you today. It's not just about dredging up the past. You begin to realize that past wounds still limit your response today.

If you practice yoga, you go beyond your ego and beyond your gender. That was appealing, but it also was an avoidance of my responsibility as a man. So many of the things Robert Bly spoke of were true for me. I was really a soft man. I would much rather do the dishes, be quiet, and play after women. I knew how to get laid, but I didn't know how to say what I felt or how to take a stand. I was afraid of my own aggression. I did not feel responsible to younger men. I didn't take responsibility for a lot of the smarmy things that our gender had done.

I have been looking for the mature elder my whole life, and I am turning into the mature elder. In India, I was talking to a young man after class. He was twenty-one and I was forty-nine. I said, "When we did shoulderstand with variations, my legs were dying." He said, "Not mine." I asked, "Are you really working your legs the whole time, or just hanging out in the poses?" He replied, "Maybe for an old man like you it's difficult, but not for me." And he didn't say that as a slap in the face, though it was a major shock for me. He said it as someone looking at someone who was middle-aged. At fifty years old, classically speaking, the householder period is over and you move on to *vanaprastha,* the forest dweller.

By no means do I think I am an old man. I don't even think of myself as an older man, except when I get around my students at DePaul University and realize I could be their father. But as I have accepted the aging process, I realize just because you are older that doesn't make you an elder. To be an elder means to take responsibility with the community. I am involved with the men's groups in Chicago. I participate in a men's conference every year. I conduct men's group meetings.

In the same way that I want to mentor in yoga, I want to mentor man-to-man in addressing emotional issues every man has. We know that men are suffering with emotional issues. A lot of men are not getting support. You don't have to solve their problems. It isn't about giving answers. It's about giving men the space to acknowledge what they feel and to overcome the general stereotype that men are not nurturing and that men hold stuff in. It's not true. We have to provide men the right environment where they can feel that they are not less of a man because these issues come up. In fact, they are more of a man.

If you associate with strong men who you respect and who have admirable qualities, and you see them fessing up to tough stuff, it invites you to do the same. You don't think of them as wimpy, because you see their shining qualities. You wouldn't think that they are weak or feminine. You see the strength in them, and yet at the same time, there's no fear to let the other side show. Strong men are not afraid of other strong men. It's like good musicians jamming. Eric Clapton doesn't have to worry about Jeff Beck upstaging him. B.B. King does his thing. They are not afraid of somebody else's creativity.

When they are jamming, it becomes a shared experience.

Absolutely.

When you get in that center where your Self is, you are not afraid of independent centers of initiative. You want to force the creativity. You don't want to shut it down. As a gender, men have not come out of posturing. We need to foster a sense of strength in ourselves and admire strength in other men. Men have to help each other. We need to be stewards of power for the good of the community. A relationship with a mentor, or an elder, is important to our personal journey. It is similar to a guru in the yoga tradition.

A guru is supposed to help you find the divine power in your own heart. A guru should give you a *mala* with your picture around your own neck. Nobody knows your way, because the uniqueness of you is like your thumbprint. Your path has never existed. It isn't preprogrammed. In fact, a lot of it is created as you walk it. You can't even know what it is, so it's as much a surprise to you as anybody else. That takes courage. That's the "follow your bliss" aspect of Joseph Campbell.

Yoga is open-ended. And not just relative to *asana*, but relative to your whole life. *Svadhyaya*, or self-study, doesn't mean just psychological introspection so you will find your personal path. It means to study the masters who have gone before. You can listen to the story of someone else's life to get a clue, but then you have to carom off that and listen to your own heart. It's your responsibility to find your way. It's also an obligation of personal power.

Do you have a mediation practice?

Pranayama practice is what has really influenced me the most in the Iyengar tradition. It's my own choice to get up earlier than the kids. They're better than alarm clocks. You know that they're going to be up between six and six-thirty every morning. Rarely I can get them to sit still in my lap while I hug them. So I try to get up earlier than them and do a little breath practice. I do not do any sitting meditation in terms of *Vipassana*, breath awareness, or *mantra* yoga. My *pranayama* practice is the closest I get to personal meditation.

I noticed that you have a lot of Native American artifacts in your yoga studio.

That's because my Jewish mother used to say, "You're a *wilde chaya* which means "wild Indian." I really try to respect all cultures. In my teaching stories, I take material from all traditions. Over the years, the wisdom of Native American traditions and rituals I have attended have influenced me. It's part of the astral migration of the United States. It's my attempt to honor letting people in community speak their peace.

I was born into a generation that realized hatred and misunderstanding of other people's religious traditions will not bring peace. Acceptance and cross-pollination of wisdom opens your heart. The Tibetan teachings were the first place where I ever read a scripture that said, "Read the scriptures of all other countries." I never found that in any other tradition. Impartially read the scriptures of all the other countries. The bee draws nectar from different flowers. Just like I want to honor the Jewish, Christian, Islamic, scientific, and artistic community, the Native American tradition has wisdom to offer.

At the same time, although I am marinated in yoga, I have come to seriously question the wholesale import of a completely other culture from another time and geography, unless it has its own American flavor. I am reminded of a story of one of the first Japanese Zen roshis to visit our country. His students went to the degree of building a temple in his honor. They constructed it with rice paper, installed sliding doors, and burnt the right incense. It was as though he had never left Japan. He told his students, "I am so thankful that you did this for me, but if you want to become enlightened, you have to be an American."

How have you used yoga for healing and what gives yoga it's healing powers?

At the physical level, strain is expensive to the body. Any time you can get rid of tension, you're in better shape. Anybody can pick up a book that says, "Lie down on your back and breath a couple of times." If you do this, you're going to feel better. But the more accurate you can be, the better the results. This is why Iyengar yoga, with its healthy alignment details and the use of the props, is as effective as anything I've seen in physical therapy. Probably more so, because it includes mental and spiritual aspects.

In the physical therapist's office, no claim is being made that you have to be morally straight as a human being. You just go on a physical level. It's not their responsibility to tell you to eat differently. They would refer you to a nutritionist. In yoga, you're buying into a certain life field that's about changing consciousness. If you change your consciousness, you change your inquiry into everything—your diet, your exercise, your lifestyle, your livelihood.

Yoga starts with the structure, but it isn't limited to just your structure. Mr. Iyengar says, "Where does the body end and the mind begin? Where does the mind end and the soul begin?" Once you see the inter-connection between these things, you're not just working on your body when you work on your body. You're working on your mind and you're working on your emotions. You can't physically take care of yourself without inquiring into your intellectual, emotional, and spiritual needs. And vice versa. Healing goes further than aligning your bones or achieving a normal blood pressure.

I worked with hospice in the mid-seventies, when Elizabeth Kübler-Ross was popularizing the movement. Part of my philosophy comes from my work with hospice. People with a terminally ill prognosis are going to die whether or not it's from cancer. There can always be a spontaneous remission, even though life is fatal. But people are not in a hospice situation until their condition is far enough advanced. They are looking for death with dignity. In other words, curing is no longer the metaphor, but you can be healed even though you die.

This is not just semantics. I have a break in a bone that is not going to be surgically repaired. I am not going to be cured from this condition. So set me on a process of learning about how to heal as much as I can. How do I not let it get me down? How do I develop the strength of my will? How do I find out if food affects me? Sugar sure does. I feel it in my joints. Does lifestyle affect me? Sure, stress does.

You broaden your approach by inquiry, by educating yourself, even if you can't cure yourself. The ideal would be that you cure yourself, and there is total disappearance of the symptom. Not just suppression, but disappearance of the symptoms. There would be healing and a new optimism that comes with it. A new enlivening, quickening quality that gives you vitality and makes you want to put yourself back into life with verve and zest. Sometimes you can't cure yourself. But the healing process can still go on by how you interact with people, how you share the lessons you learn, and how you help others.

Where do you see your life evolving? What are you striving for every day?

I have to admit, I don't think I'm striving. At one point, I was like the person pumping the handle on the well. I really had to pump hard because the water was down three hundred feet. By pumping sufficiently, I got the flow going and now I don't have to pump that same way I did then. I can give it an easy rocking motion and keep the flow going. I don't want to be overreacting to the word "striving," and sound like I am perfectly at peace and there are no challenges in my life. But in a broad sense, I don't see myself struggling to reach something that I don't think I have acquired.

I like to think of life as unfolding. Where is it leading? I don't know where it's leading. That's the mystery of being. I joke with my wife about it. When you marry somebody, you come together with someone who is completely other than you, even though initially there are so many things that resonate. You feel you are kindred spirits. But as you get on with your relationship, one of the things you realize about allowing the person to be other than you, is that they are other than the way you want them to be. And so is life.

Every day in our relationship is another day of history. I've never gone this far with any woman in my life before. Whatever is going on with my children has never happened before. That brings a certain freshness, because it's unfolding. There is a constant reminder of how it's all happening, and it's never happened before.

I want to do a good job as a dad. My children's happiness and their positive perception of me are important, and I don't want to do anything to tarnish that. At the same time, I don't want the life my wife and I have together to solely revolve around earning a livelihood and providing for our kids. When does life begin? The Catholic says, "It begins at conception." The Protestant says, "It begins when the heart starts beating." The Jewish guy says, "When the kids finally graduate." I look forward to another stage of life that will come to my wife and I. Even though we have consciously chosen to build a family, we both talk about another stage in our life that we are looking forward to.

I would like to see the yoga studio become strong enough to run on its own, so that the power of my personality isn't what draws the majority of students. I would like to see the younger teachers become creative powers so that the school runs on the power of yoga. I would like to continue to mentor young men and help make an impact on their lives.

Other than that, I don't have a lot of big, worldwide plans. I will just continue to let my life unfold. I have had some uncanny success with following the inner voice at different times of my life. The next time the inner voice speaks, hopefully, I will be listening and follow whatever it tells me at that moment.

Gabriel Halpern holds an M.A. in Health Psychology and a B.A. in Philosophy. He received Iyengar yoga certification from at the institutes in San Francisco and Pune, India. He has studied and taught since 1970. An accomplished vegetarian chef and practitioner of kitchen sink mysticism, Gabriel loves cooking for relatives and friends. Gabriel embodies the yoga of family and relationship with his wife, Margaret, and their prides and joys, Tara and Kailey. Gabriel is known for his enthusiasm, clarity, precision, compassion, and zany sense of humor. He inspires people to feed from the treasures of Eastern wisdom, while at the same time being true to their own path as a Western and contemporary practitioner.

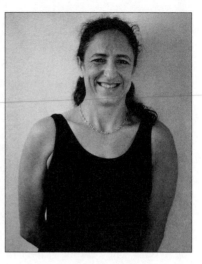

GABRIELLA GIUBILARO
FLORENCE, ITALY

How did you come to teach in America?

I came to assist my teacher, Dona Holleman, when she came to the states. I did it every single summer for many years, and it was very helpful for me. I assisted her in the states, Holland, and Switzerland. For any person who wants to learn to teach, it is really important to be an assistant and help in a class. When you're in an apprenticeship and helping, you have more time to observe. When you're teaching, you're busy with everybody in the class. I have been very lucky that I had the opportunity to assist classes for many, many years, learning how to touch, how to watch, and how to help.

When I decided not to assist my teacher anymore, and I said good-bye to everybody, they asked me, "Why don't you come by yourself?" The first year I said, "No." When I came back to Italy, I said to myself, "Why not? I'm not working in the summer anyway, so why not go and try? If can pay my expenses, maybe I can see new places." I went to small places, where there were not any big centers, to help the local people do Iyengar yoga. For many years, I went every summer to work with the same teachers and groups. That was always my mentality—to go, to work, and to help people who needed it.

What was your introduction to yoga?

I read *The Autobiography of a Yogi* by Paramahansa Yogananda when I was twenty-two years old, and I thought it was interesting. A cousin from Sicily gave it to me as a present. I told myself, "I'm never going to do any yoga in Italy, because I'm sure there is not any serious teacher." I thought either I could do it in a serious way or forget about it. I could only learn from someone who was a very serious teacher, not a person who was a *dilettante*. I don't understand why people study yoga or even how to cook from a person who knows a little bit. I can only study with people who really know what they are doing and what they are teaching. I demand that from a teacher. I can't understand people who don't choose the most qualified teacher. That's not my way.

I went to visit some American friends in Florence and they said, "We're going out to a yoga class. There is a teacher who is very good." I said, "I'll come with you." I went in ski clothes and full underwear. Only the fingers were out. My toes, feet, and neck were completely covered. It was really ridiculous. I liked it and went back the next week. I was very impressed, because my teacher, Dona Holleman, would say, "Spread your toes." I didn't even know you could move your toes. I was so surprised by the idea of elongating each toe of the foot and lifting the ankle of the foot. I was so surprised at this methodical philosophy, this precision of each movement. It was like a new world. Like a miracle.

I continued once a week for one year. Then I decided to work a little bit more and do it twice a week. Every time we did something in class I could not do, I would go home and try. I was practicing almost every day, because I did not understand why I could not do something. I had a strong practice from the beginning, but a very strange practice. After four years, Dona asked me if I wanted to teach, and I did. I was much happier than when I finished my studies and started to work. I was enjoying teaching, but I didn't have big expectations. My interest and the energy I was putting into it grew slowly over the years.

What were you studying at the university?

Physics. My idea was to do research at the university and maybe to teach. I worked for one year at the university doing research part-time. When you finish your studies in Italy, it's not so easy to have a job at the university. When I was studying physics, I had this idea that I had to give all my energy to do the best I could do. I wasn't thinking about getting money or power, only doing my best.

In the beginning, I put all my time, energy, and effort into studying physics. Slowly, the interest in physics decreased and the interest in yoga increased. Then I found my energy was divided. I realized it was too much to try to put one foot in yoga and one foot in the university. I knew I had to choose.

In 1978, I did both—teaching yoga and working at the university. That was a lucky coincidence, because I could experiment with both. Society respects much more a person who is a professor at a university, and this was very important to my family. Everybody was expecting I would go on in my studies and in my work, including my family. My parents couldn't understand why I chose yoga. It was completely out of their mentality.

Was it difficult to choose yoga?

Yes, because of their expectations. I was teaching once a week and I had no idea if I could be a good yoga teacher. Yoga was not popular at all in Italy. I had four students. My heart was telling me to teach yoga and my brain was telling me to stay at the university. One day, I told myself if I don't run the risk and try to teach yoga, later in life I would regret it. If I couldn't teach yoga, at least I would know I tried. I thought it was important to follow my heart.

I decided to teach yoga, even if I ended up selling clothes in a shop. I did this part-time when I was a teenager, and it was very boring. The women would put dresses on and say, "How do I look?" I had no idea what to say, because they looked awful. I knew I was supposed to say, "You look great!" But I couldn't do it.

"This dress makes you look thin." That's always another good one.

It's funny. We all have our little nightmares. This friend of mine said, "I need to go away for five days. Can you go and work for me in this shop?" I had just had an accident with a scooter and my foot was broken. I had plaster from my ankle up to my knee, and I was limping. There I was in one of the most elegant shops in the center of Florence with women wanting me to help them get dressed.

What have you been able to bring from your university studies, especially physics, into yoga instruction?

A lot of things. First of all, if you study science you have a different approach, a different mentality. We learn how to observe in the scientific mind, and it's completely different from the philosophical mind and the psychological mind. We have a different approach to studying an existing situation. If I explain something in class, I have to be very methodical. I can't jump from one thing to another thing without a link or without a connection. I can't say something that contradicts something I said before. If there is any contradiction, I explain why. People who don't have a mathematical mentality jump from idea to idea without a link, without a connection, and without clarity.

Another thing that comes from my studies is the understanding of the *asanas*. Physics is both dynamic and static. Every time I do a movement, or teach a movement, I know the laws of the dynamic and the laws of the static. I remember these laws inside myself, even if I don't express this in the class, because it would be too difficult for the student to understand. It's helped me to have a very simple depiction of all of the *asanas*.

What changes did you experience when you started yoga?

In the beginning, nothing. I only know I was surprised at discovering my own body. I had no idea that you could think with the body. That was my wonder, my surprise, and my discovery. Before starting yoga, I had already stopped smoking and drinking coffee and wine, because I discovered that it was not good for my health. So I can see I had some kind of connection with my body. But when reading some article about vegetarians, I remember thinking it was only a religious thing.

Anything that had to do with metaphysical energy was only a strange idea of people who were a little bit out of their mind. And it took me many, many years of practicing yoga before I started to believe. Even to believe a tree is all energy took me many, many years of work on myself. To me, energy was only dynamic and potential. I was not the kind of person who would read a book and believe. I was very skeptical.

What caused the paradigm shift for you?

My practice. What happens with practice is you go from the gross body to the subtle body. When you are in the gross body, you can see only gross things, gross experiences. As you go inside, you can observe and believe in more subtle experiences.

As the body opens up, your mind opens up. The biggest change I started to see was that I felt much more connected with nature. Before I was not aware at all of saving energy or any ecological problems. I started to be more interested and aware of it. I started buying different kinds of soap, and different kinds of products I was using in the house. I started being careful about saving energy, because I was becoming more connected.

I grew up in a city. I could go to the country and to the beach only in the summer. I would spend one month at the beach and one month in the country. After I started to do yoga, I started to discover the flowers and the trees. I moved to the country and really started to discover the seasons. It was a surprise to see how the leaves would change color and then fall down. When the spring would come, I would notice what came first. In some trees, the flowers came first and then the leaves. Other trees started with the leaves. I began to observe, to watch, and to discover all these new worlds. I am sure this comes from my yoga practice.

I became more aware of what I was eating. I became vegetarian three years after I started to do yoga—and not out of decision. It came by itself.

In life, we mix food with our emotional mind. Our emotional mind tells us what to eat and not to eat. If I am nervous, if I am upset, if something is bothering me, if I am unhappy, or if I don't have love, I will go into the kitchen and eat. Some people don't eat. At the table, you eat because you have company. Reading books about diet is our mental body. Intellectually we decide what we want. The mind does not know what the body needs. If you discover the intelligence of your body, eating becomes much simpler.

You need to give way to the intelligence of the body, and the intelligence of the body doesn't come in one day. If you are used to eating chocolate every day, the body will tell you, "I want chocolate." If you are used to drinking coffee, your body will tell you, "I want coffee." That is not the intelligence of the body. That's only habits. The body goes with habits. If I do yoga every morning, when I wake up in the morning, my body wants to do yoga. But if I don't do it every day, then I have to push myself to do yoga. The body gets habits very easily. That's why it's better to do yoga every day at the same time, because it comes much easier.

To get intelligence of the body for the food, you need to break habits slowly. But once you awaken this intelligence, the body can tell you what to eat and what not to eat. I am very happy when I sit in front of a plate of salad. Really! I enjoy it! I am very happy I am going to eat it. I don't remember being like that before. Never. I can't remember being happy in front of any plate before I started practicing yoga. If I have some vegetables, some greens, some grains, I am very happy. I enjoy it. And not because I am telling myself, "This is good for me."

Coming from a scientific background and being skeptical of the metaphysical, was it hard for you to develop a meditation practice?

When I started yoga classes, I would do the *pranayama*. It was through the *pranayama* that I started to have a meditation practice. I really believe what Iyengar says—there is no division between *pranayama* and meditation, if you do *pranayama* in the right way. I believe it, because I experienced it. The meditation comes by itself, if I practice *pranayama* in the right way. If I don't have enough time, I prefer to do *pranayama*, because I think it's much more powerful than any other practice. If I don't practice *pranayama* in the morning, I feel the difference in the rest of the day. If I practice *asanas* in the right way, there is no difference between meditation and *asanas*. The only meditation is to meditate with all of your body—the physical, mental, and psychological body.

If I don't do *pranayama*, I am irritable during the day, and I can get out of balance easily. If I have done a good practice, nothing can touch me during the day. I feel much more centered, grounded. I have a deep connection inside myself. There's a core inside that nobody can touch. It's such a nice feeling, because no matter what happens around me, I am always in touch with this part of myself that is beyond the physical. *Pranayama* gives clarity of the mind. If I have a good practice of *pranayama,* it gives this sharpness of the mind that is impossible to describe.

I am not saying that meditation is only *pranayama,* but I am saying that *pranayama* done in the right way is the same as meditation. In the beginning, *pranayama* was just a breathing technique. In the beginning, it is this way for almost everybody. With Iyengar, I really learned how to be present with the breath and not just to count. I started to not be worried about how long was my breath, how long was the inhalation and the exhalation, but to be more in the present and to work more with the connection of the body and the mind.

Describe your first experience with India.

I went to India ten years after I had started practicing yoga. I had already met Iyengar in Holland. I stayed there for three months. It was a shock in the beginning. Just to be in the airport in Bombay was a shock. It was the first time I ever went to a really poor country.

In India, they still practice a culture that developed thousands of years ago. India is absolutely a different culture from Europe. How they eat is different. How they behave socially is different. Everything is different from Europe.

I was staying in a Christian nun *ashram*. It was a very nice place in Pune, close to the institute where I would go and study with Iyengar. I was not in a real Indian environment, but it was a very warm feeling.

I was shocked at the class. Iyengar was not teaching classes, but he continued to teach intensives. He was in the class. He was helping when he wanted. He was interrupting when he wanted, so I still had the experience of his personality.

And that was a shock?

Yes. He has a very strong personality. When he is close to you, no matter what *asana* you are doing, you have to do your best. He doesn't even need to touch you. The first month I had so much fear that I could not do much. I couldn't even sleep at night. When I started to relax when he was close to me, I learned how to give more of myself. Even if at that moment I thought I was doing my best, when he was there, I could do more. I learned to break my limitation and to go beyond it.

This is what I really liked about Iyengar. I could see he puts his heart in the class. He puts all his passion, all his love, all his care, and all his energy to get the maximum of what any student can do in that moment. In class, he puts all his fire that comes from the passion that is inside. He is like a volcano that can't hold it in. And it's great. Once you go beyond the fear, it's really wonderful to see him teaching, to see his eyes, and to see what he can do with any person.

Is your goal to bring that same passion to your teaching?

It's my goal in teaching, but it could be misunderstood, because you cannot copy another person. I am very concerned to see how many other teachers try to copy Iyengar. There is no way to copy Iyengar, like there is no way to copy anyone. The more I understand myself, the more I can understand others. The more I awaken the intelligence of my body, the more I can awaken the intelligence of others. My goal is to follow his example, not to copy him. I really think he is a genius in what he has done. To be a healer, you need to know how to heal yourself. He has been a genius in understanding his body. Not only the physical body, but also the psychological body and the mental body.

Did you find him warm outside of the class setting?

He was very warm, and that was another shock. When I was there, the Iyengars were organizing a trip outside of Pune. We went to see some villages and a river in a holy place. Outside the class, Iyengar was so nice and easy to talk to. He joked and laughed. He was like a child. I was impressed at this behavior outside the class. In the class, he was a leader. He was really strong and powerful—so strong, you felt like he was in another dimension. You couldn't even go close to him. When we were outside the class, he was the most normal, loving, and joking person.

You eventually opened your own studio.

Just a few years before my mother died, she thought I needed my own place where I could work, because she was afraid if I was teaching in different places, I wouldn't have any security in my life. She bought a small apartment for me and even paid for some renovations, so now I have this very small yoga room. It's full with twelve people. If it happens that we have sixteen people, we really have to be very precise with the sticky mats.

For many years my mother was completely against the yoga. She was a wonderful mother, but she would tell everybody I had passed from physics to physical education. When my mother died, I discovered nobody knew I was teaching yoga! She thought yoga was a religious thing.

Are there any major differences between European yoga and American yoga?

The main difference I find between the Americans and Europeans is that in American yoga, people are much more open, friendly, easygoing, and quicker to accept new ideas and new things. They get enthusiastic very easily. Because of this openness, they can say, "I want to do yoga for the rest of my life." And after one week, they have forgotten because something else new has come along.

European people are not so easygoing, not so open to new ideas, systems, methods, and teachers. But once they start to know a system and a teacher, they are much more grounded and faithful. If they decide they want to do yoga, it's usually a deeper decision than in an American person.

Do you think the dynamic growth of yoga in America is a fad?

I don't think so anymore. Yoga has been here for enough years.

There is a big movement in teachers developing their own way—moving away from the tradition, taking from different traditions, and following their own paths. For example, some people mix *ashtanga* yoga with Iyengar yoga. Personally, I do not like to mix the two. We need so many years of polishing our bodies before we come to a real intelligence of the body. I try to follow what Iyengar says and what he teaches. I don't invent my own stuff. A lot of people say that this is rigidity of mind, but I don't think it's rigidity of mind. Within this system there is still so much variety, I don't feel stuck. But in my variety, I still follow Iyengar's guidelines. Of course, no matter how much we try to follow a system or a teacher, we always filter in our personalities.

There are so many systems sprouting, but I am not interested in a new system of yoga. I want to see what I can learn from Iyengar and profit from his knowledge as much as I can. This is important, not only for me, but it is ethical in relation to my students. Even if I am filtering with my personality, I try to preserve the understanding and the knowledge of the person I respect and trust.

At the same time, the world is big enough to have a place for everybody. I admire people who have the courage to follow their own path. Their *karma* is taking them.

Where is your karma *taking you?*

I will continue to teach yoga as long as my heart is there. I hope it never becomes work.

Gabriella Giubilaro was born in Palermo, Sicily and grew up in Florence, Italy, where she attended college and received a Ph.D. in Physics. She began the practice of yoga at the age of twenty-three under the tutelage of Dona Holleman and began teaching five years later. After a decade of practice, Gabriella traveled to Pune, India to study yoga with B.K.S. Iyengar; his daughter, Geeta; and his son, Prashant. Since her initial visit to Pune, she has returned annually to study with the Iyengars. She has translated *Light on Yoga Sutras of Patanjali* by B.K.S. Iyengar into Italian. Gabriella is the director of the Light on Yoga Association Italy yoga studio in Florence and conducts workshops in the United States and Eastern Europe.

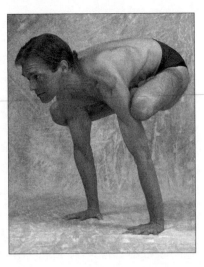

RICHARD FREEMAN
BOULDER

You tell a wonderful story about Tibetan monks that I love. It's a great lesson in religious tolerance.

A number of years ago, there was a group of Tibetan monks going to different fine art museums around the country putting on a show of their art. One of their arts is the creation of very large sand *mandalas*, which are exquisite sand paintings of minute detail. There is a very fine ritual in creating them. They chant *mantras* while they are laying down the borders and creating sacred space. It's quite concentrated work that takes days.

People will come to the museum to see the monks working and hear them chanting. One fellow came and apparently didn't like it very much. He considered them to be a bunch of heathens mumbling Satan's name. He was very threatened by the *mandala,* because it was a symbol opposing his symbols. He identified with his symbols. He went running into a nearly completed *mandala,* kicked it, and scattered it across the room while screaming about the devil. The monks started laughing. Amazingly, they weren't upset at all. This irate and irrationally religious man was trying to destroy their intricate and sacred creation. Part of the ritual, after the monks complete the *mandala* and it sits for a while, is that they destroy it and sweep it all off in dustpans. The sacred space is erased.

Truth is conveyed through forms, but the forms dissolve. We humans get very attached to the shape of the container that truth is being delivered in—the style of the church, the shape of the crucifix, the particular story or myth. We identify something temporary with the truth, even though it's only functioning as a metaphor for or an expression of truth. The religious form needs to be periodically dropped in order to directly experience the present moment—raw, unstructured, and open.

The ego grabs on to form, and the form becomes an ornament of the ego. It makes you feel certain and secure, so that you are not facing raw consciousness. But God is pure consciousness, not an object. Intelligence is a waking up from mental creations and fantasies, so that when awake, we have no structured position to defend. Allow criticism to come. It can really only refine our understanding. Having insight into how religious forms and practices work in producing mystical experience, we can be more relaxed. As a Buddhist might say, "Intelligence is seeing emptiness in any form."

When did you discover yoga?

I first discovered yoga in 1963 when I was thirteen years old. It was actually Thoreau who opened my eyes. Emerson, Thoreau, and the early American transcendentalists were the first people in this country to get translations of the *Upanishads* and the *Bhagavad Gita.*

Thirteen is a young age to be reading Thoreau. I was still reading The Hardy Boys.

Thoreau's *Walden* was one of the first real books I read. I found it in my older sister's stuff. It really captured my heart and put me into another state. I loved reading about forests, detailed descriptions of nature, and the present moment, especially at that young age. I became interested in reading philosophy, which was extracurricular at my high school. I would often skip lunch and go to the library to read Kant and Hegel, and try to make sense of it. I was a bit of an oddball.

I'm going to say you weren't dating material.

Oh, I wasn't typical. Though none of my friends were interested in so-called "normal" cultural rituals either. My high school experience was during the sixties, and there were some very different ideas and radical transformations beginning then.

I went off to a college in northwestern Illinois, which had been started as an experiment in original source learning in the fifties. By 1968, it was known as a school for experiment in alternative awareness. It was an opportunity for me to explore my interest in mysticism, philosophy, and yoga practices. I studied Taoism, Buddhism, and yoga. I began to practice yoga and meditation for hours, while floating on the spirit of the times.

Did psychedelics open you up to insight and wisdom you might not have otherwise experienced?

I experienced passionate insight or spirit before I ever considered experimenting with anything to help me along. Using a psycho-active agent is like being booted into orbit. Those types of experi-ences bring along with them subtle illusions. Rarely someone will experience some insight while intoxicated. They then might give the credit to the intoxicant. You might experience spirit or salt while intoxicated, because there is nothing but salt or spirit anyway. Such experiences are artificial because they play with our body chemistry so much that a great imbalance and fatigue occur, and you start interpreting the experience incorrectly.

As humans, we identify the spiritual part of an experience with the content of the mind. Having positive associations with the con-tent, we try to repeat the content rather than the context. If we had insight into context, we would allow anything to become an object of meditation, to be sacred. Instead, we see only the content of the mind, which is a particular vision like a flower or a pretty pattern, and we think, "That's what I want." The symbol becomes the thing. People do that with drugs as well as without. We associate all of these things with a mystical experience, and by doing so, go off into all sorts of fantasies.

As we become awakened through yoga, we can see the gap between what really is happening and such fantasies. We see the suffering that comes from such misunderstandings, and we pay clos-er attention our minds.

I would speculate you were a philosophy major.

Exactly. I fit right in.

Were you involved in a yoga community in college?

I had friends who were meditators. I would sometimes go to the Chicago Zen Center for instruction and community. There was support for meditation and mystical practices in general, but for yoga practice in particular, there was very little. Wanting to go deep into practice, I left college in 1970 with the intention to live at Tassajara Zen Mountain Center. En route, I met a Krishna devotee and, instead of in a Zen community, I wound up living in a small Krishna *ashram* with three others. It was actually very pleasant. They were not into proselytizing and syrupy sweet fundamentalism. There was real sincerity and mysticism. Yet the Krishna practices soon started to become a movement.

Then there came a twist in the teachings, which was the taking of this beautiful yogic myth of Radha and Krishna and literalizing it into historical fact—God looks like this, Krishna is the best *mantra*, etc. Then came the preaching and the jamming of it down everyone's throat. As soon as this started to happen, I decided to go.

And you didn't want to sell roses on street corners.

They, like any fundamentalist group, specialized in putting others down. They had major trouble with Buddhism, with *Advaita Vedanta*, with classical yoga, with Christianity, with Islam, with all forms of modern science, and even with other Krishna branches in India. I guess that might happen with any group, based on doctrine. One day, they even insulted Bach. I grew up on Bach. This was an eye opener for me. No one insults Bach.

And gets away with it!

I went to India and after an intricate journey wound up in Vrindavana, which is the "holy land" of Krishna's play. Everything there is considered sacred, even the rocks, dust, and trees. It is a ritualized place full of *ashrams*, temples, and *sadhus*. I stayed there not quite a year. I became a *sannyasin*, taking a vow of renunciation. I separated myself from the Krishna organization, any organization for that matter, and started to travel with a friend. It always helps to have a friend when you are off adventuring.

What did you renounce?

That's a good question. I believe that the renunciation is an internal state in which even one's thoughts, feelings, and sensations are perceived to be sacred, to be *shakti*, to be God's, to be vibrating *prana*. What to speak of external things and other beings. They too should not be reduced to being objects of our ego. However, in its commonly understood meaning, renunciation is a monastic inten- tion in which you minimize your possessions. The order in India was at one time highly respected. Socially, it involves being willing to teach in exchange for food and temporary shelter. It's not a bad exchange, if the *sannyasi* has something to teach. Often it is just a welfare system for those who don't like to work.

So, for some time I traveled in India, presenting my rather limit- ed perspective on life and yoga. People were so kind to me and so thrilled that a Westerner loved yoga. I did a lot of traveling in south- east Asia. Once in Bengal, I met an Iranian friend, who invited me to come to Iran to teach yoga. I went, and to my surprise, I really loved the place. The culture and the people were beautiful. There were deep traditions of esoteric, spiritual practice woven into every- day things. The food, by the way, was excellent, too.

My friend had an excellent set up in Tehran, and his cousin became the first yoga student. He was a devout Sufi and a fine gen- tleman. All the first yoga students were Sufis or people from the diplomatic community. Gradually, people from all strata of society came for yoga. Most people were already conversant in some sort of spiritual tradition, which required that I become a translator of the inner experiences of yoga from Hindu images to Islamic metaphors on to psychological explanation. I felt something like I imagine Spinoza felt, being able to disguise one religion within another, within another, and so on.

I was exposed deeply to Iranian culture and enjoyed myself tremendously. I could pass for a Muslim, having learned verses from the Koran. When people found out that I was an American, they said, "Wow!" They were so happy and open once they got over the initial fear of the "other." Politics and religion divide people, though they are intended to unite them.

What was your motivation in coming back to the states?

There was a revolution occurring in Iran that was getting to be quite bloody and dangerous. I thought it would be prudent to get out of there.

Was the hostage crisis occurring at that time?

No, the revolution was beginning to form. That was before the hostage crisis and before the government fell. The royal family had left, except for the Shah and the Queen. There were great riots and demonstrations which would end up as bloody conflicts with the army. It was becoming quite dangerous to be there, especially as a foreigner. An opportunity came to leave, so I left. After traveling through Europe, I wound up back at my parent's home and they were glad to see me. I was twenty-eight-and-a-half and coming full circle, through different cultures and religions, back to the nest opened my eyes.

Was there a decompression period when you returned?

Oh, yeah.

Did you have a newfound appreciation for America?

I kissed the ground.

America is a great place. It has some problem areas, but the free, secular, democratic, multicultural structure is the best for real spiritual awakening. Here ideas are synthesized. America allows its citizens to criticize it. This is rare, but it allows continuous growth and adaptation. Many governments around the world and many religious traditions won't allow criticism.

In the Western yoga world and in the New Age movement, critical thinking is also unfortunately rare. Can we learn to examine our own presuppositions? Can we see how our beliefs, hopes, and our thinking are structured? Through self-reflection and self-criticism, thinking evolves. You need to have intensity and insight into thought to be a mystic. Otherwise, you will be living in self-deception. You must doubt ideas and look at them to get to their roots. Such critical thinking is not negative thinking. It is intelligence free of fear.

When you came back from Iran were you committed to teaching yoga?

I was committed to finding the radical, underlying truth of the mystical experience, free of religious beliefs and dogma—to finding what sort of practice, if any, could invite or induce that experience—so that I could be free of self-deception. When I first came back, I didn't do any practice for a month. I traveled around, visited with friends, and read philosophy. I settled down in Boulder and became a plumber for four months. I wanted to experience a blue-collar job that was just plain old work. I was pretty good at plumbing and plumbing language, which is a special style of cursing that plumbers use like magical *mantras* to get pipes to fit together. It was nice to come back to a simple life.

Did you find great wisdom in that experience?

Yeah, that I didn't want to be a plumber!

Did you go to trade school?

No, there was an old plumber looking for an assistant. He couldn't figure out why I wanted to do this. He said, "What's a fellow like you want to do plumbing for?" I said, "Well, it's a challenge."

Were you a vegetarian plumber?

Oh, yes. A truck full of hay once went by and my boss said, "There goes Richard's lunch! Ha, ha, ha!" He instead would have six beers for lunch.

What would you pack in your lunch box?

I would have a tofu sandwich and carrots.

I'm seeing a sitcom—"The Yogi and the Plumber." A contemporary version of "Chico and the Man." This could be big.

Yoga is good for plumbing, because you have to crawl into awkward places and get under sinks. If you're flexible, you have a great advantage. Plumbing involves finding the plumb line, so does yoga.

Were you flexible prior to yoga?

I was fairly flexible. My forward bending wasn't good. My back bending was fair. I've had to work many hours for years to become supple. In my early teens, I practiced gymnastics in which the focus was only strength and coordination.

Were you an ashtanga *yoga practitioner in Iran?*

No, not an *ashtanga vinyasa* practitioner. I had started studies with an Iyengar teacher in Tehran. She was from Bombay and was married to an Iranian businessman. She held classes in her living room for her Iranian friends and people in the Indian community. She was very gracious, but the level of intensity and mysticism did not impress me. I would just roll my eyes. Then she invited an older Iyengar student from Bombay to Tehran for a workshop. I got a good dose, and it started to influence me. I gradually started to understand and incorporate Iyengar yoga into what I was doing.

Did you study with Iyengar?

Yes, but not in India. Later I studied with him when he was in the states on different teaching trips. I have had a good connection with him. My learning style is that I will go and see or hear something, and then from that seed I can digest and extract a tremendous amount of information. I learn best that way, rather than sequentially building. I still continue to pick up gems from Mr. Iyengar and from his students.

When did you discover ashtanga *yoga?*

I didn't hear about it until after I left Iran and was living in Boulder. I had read Deshikachar's writings and was incorporating the *vinyasa* principles into my practice before I heard about Pattabhi Jois. I wanted more intensity, focus, and vigor, and I sensed there was great potential in sequencing the advanced poses. There was a smooth, cool fire.

I met Pattabhi Jois at the Feathered Pipe Ranch in 1987. We had a deep and intuitive connection. I had studied Sanskrit, and he tuned right into that. I could understand what he was talking about. One of the difficulties with the *ashtanga* tradition is that Pattabhi Jois doesn't speak much English. Context and nuance are difficult to transmit solely with the eyebrows. Precise language and ideas are helpful. Pattabhi Jois is very much intent on philosophy, chanting, and meditation. He won't teach them unless you, too, are intent on them.

After meeting Pattahbi Jois, my wife and I went to Mysore to study with him for six months. That was our first stint. For about a month, we were the only students there. What great luck we had! I could spend hours asking him questions. He would quote verse after verse. Usually, I could recognize the subject matter and could research the original texts later. He taught *pranayama*, *mudra*, and meditation. I really quizzed him about *mulabandha*. He explained the *ashtanga* system to me as an internal system, making clear its purpose.

Which is?

It's yoga. It transmutes the body, the senses, the nervous system, the heart, and the mind until everything, inside and out, is perceived as spirit. The *asana* and *pranayama* practice opens the energy channels including the central *nadi*, the *sushumna*. Drawing the internal breath into it leads into *samadhi*, and on through into self-knowledge. I don't think its purpose is ego enhancement, although you have to start somewhere.

Describe your regimen in Mysore.

On our first trip to Mysore, I did primary series the first day. The second day I was there, I did the intermediate or second series.

The third day I was there, I started the third series. I spent two months on the third series, and then started the forth series.

When learning third series, I would do both the first series and second series, and then work on the third, all in one session. When I completed third, I would do first and third one day, and second and third the next day, gradually adding on the forth series one or two poses at a time. After finishing forth, I would practice half of one of the first two series for warm up, then all of the third and forth every day. So that made four different warm up routines before the advanced postures. I was creamed. But cream is sweet. It's nectar.

How long did that take?

Four hours a day.

In one session?

Yeah. A big sweat bath. A big puddle on the floor.

Wow!

Then after an hour rest, I would do *pranayama* for forty-five minutes. This was all just on the initial six months in Mysore. Each subsequent trip has been different and challenging.

Please tell me you were struggling.

I was struggling as I learned. Sometimes I was struggling from fatigue. I would get tweaked now and then. My shoulder would get sore. I once tore an intercostal muscle. Nothing major, but aches and pains would come and go. I never indulged them. I kept improving my alignment. When breath and alignment are present, there is no struggle.

Did you know all of the postures?

Some of them were new. Because of the way they are sequenced, all of a sudden you can do a pose you haven't done before.

Were you doing this six days a week?

Some weeks, depending on holidays. You would pray for holidays.

Describe your practice today.

I have less time than I would like for formal practice. Being a parent, a teacher, running a yoga studio, and traveling take an enormous amount of time. An important part of my practice is sitting, chanting, and *pranayama*. Two or three times a week I get to do full series practice. Otherwise, I take what I get, just trying to take the thread, the essence of the yoga throughout the day.

Yet you have maintained your flexibility.

Pretty much. I can do most of the posture fairly easily. I can't spend all of my time on *asanas*, since I need to respond to the needs of other people. Being a householder, relationship becomes a large factor in everything. We have to work more efficiently in the *asanas*.

Is there a sixth series?

There is, but it is practically a mythological series. Pattabhi Jois has it written in an old notebook. I don't know if I want to learn it. Fifth series is challenging enough. No one to my knowledge does it.

Perhaps at one point Pattabhi Jois could do all of the series. Presently, he does meditation, *pranayama*, and chants. To my knowledge, that's all he does for practice, then he teaches vigorously for five to six hours most every day. He's a great yogi and an amazing powerhouse.

What are your thoughts concerning ashtanga *yoga being a five thousand-year-old tradition that was rediscovered?*

I don't think the actual specific series are, but that sounds like good packaging. The internal methodology of *ashtanga* yoga could be 5,000 years old. The *Rig Veda*, which is that old, has references to longhaired sages, and is full of esoteric hymns about deep mystical states and yogic principles. I don't know if it was termed yoga then.

Is ashtanga *yoga the genius of Pattabhi Jois?*

Yes and no. Krishnamacharya was the synthesizer of different strands of practice and, to my knowledge, composed the specific series in detail. Pattabhi Jois has specialized in them and has refined them. However, the *vinyasa* methodology has old scriptural references. Historical study in India is always shrouded in some mystery, so you're never sure whether you have fact or myth.

Did you know Krishnamacharya?

No. That would have been quite an experience. I have learned a lot from Krishnamacharya's teaching. I read anything that comes out of the school in Madras. I try to incorporate the principles of *viniyoga* into the *ashtanga* system, so I can include more people. I also bring in Iyengar yoga—the principles of alignment and detailed attention—into doing *ashtanga* yoga. I have studied Buddhist *Vipas-*

sana meditation, as well as Zen. I bring both of those into yoga. I also bring in Sufism. It just makes yoga work better.

When did you start teaching the ashtanga practice?

I started teaching after the first week with Pattabhi Jois at Feathered Pipe Ranch. I didn't force everyone into the first series, but I taught them the principles, as I understood them. We worked on the series, fairly intelligently, so people weren't getting injured. After I went to India, he certified me as a teacher.

Are there many certified ashtanga teachers in America?

There are about five or six people around the world that I know of who are certified. Pattabhi Jois likes for people to complete the forth series before he certifies them. He likes to put them through the mill, so they experience physical transformation, if not transformation deep in their hearts. People ask him about teaching and he says, "Twelve years of practice, completing the advanced series, then teaching is possible." He's concerned about people not knowing what the purpose of the series is. I think he is correct in that. There is much misrepresentation of what *ashtanga* yoga actually is. It is a meditative and refined method. Knowing it internally, you can adapt to the individual in a non-violent and non-mechanical way. Just knowing the order of the series and the superficial geometry of the poses is like knowing only the skin of a sweet fruit.

How had becoming a householder changed your practice?

It's a real challenge to take the situation of having a family and to do it as yogically as possible. You can't have your family do yoga all day, especially children. They're not interested in that. They're struggling with the basics of growing up. Staying balanced requires you to see all things as sacred, because occasionally you miss your practice. You have got to be present and mindful of all the other things. That's the challenge—to have a balanced, real life. If you do that then your yoga practice becomes quite easy. The hardest series is nothing compared to real life.

Richard Freeman has been a student of yoga since 1968. He has spent nearly nine years in Asia studying various traditions, which he incorporates into the *ashtanga* yoga practice taught by his principal teacher, K. Pattabhi Jois of Mysore, India. His background includes Zen and *Vipassana* Buddhist practice, *Bhakti,* traditional hatha yoga, and Sufism. Since 1974, he has studied Iyengar yoga. He is an avid student of Western and Eastern philosophy, as well as Sanskrit. His ability to juxtapose various viewpoints, without losing the depth and integrity of each, has helped Richard develop a unique, metaphorical teaching style. He lives with his family in Boulder, Colorado where he directs the Yoga Workshop.

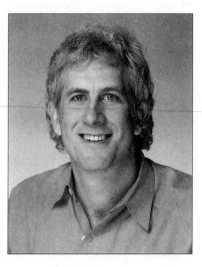

JOHN FRIEND
HOUSTON

How did you become a yoga teacher?

My yoga teacher got very sick and asked me to substitute. After that experience, I taught a weekly class through college. I graduated from Texas A&M in 1983 and taught one class a week until 1986, when I started teaching two classes a week.

After college, I went into finance and accounting. It was a successful endeavor, but it wasn't giving me the sense of fulfillment that my two yoga classes a week were giving me. I didn't want my epitaph to read, "He made a lot of money, but he didn't help much." In my heart, I couldn't handle that, because the most important thing for me was to help people.

In 1987, I made a commitment to teach yoga full-time. I didn't

know how I was going to do it, but I quit my consulting job in
Ohio, got in my car, and drove across the country to California. I
didn't have any plans or know where I was going. One afternoon, I
stopped in the middle of nowhere. I was completely unattached. It
was the first time in my life I felt totally free. I knew yoga was going
to be the thing for me. After six months in California of driving
around and taking classes, I moved back to Texas and started teaching full-time.

How did the California yoga classes influence you?

I started doing Iyengar yoga during my travels to California. I
had heard the Iyengar style was tough, but I didn't know too much
about it. I decided to go to the Iyengar Institute in San Francisco
and take a class. Since I was already teaching yoga, I thought I was
advanced, so I looked for the hardest class. The level 4 & 5
teacher's class was on Friday mornings with Judith Lasater. The
schedule said to call the teacher for permission. I called Judith and
explained that I was a yoga teacher from Texas. I didn't say I had
never done Iyengar yoga before, I just asked for permission to
attend the class. She said I was welcome to come.

Judith proceeded to give a strong class, and I was totally blown
away. I was muscling the poses, trying to maintain any sense of dignity I had left. One pose sticks in my mind—*parivrtta trikonasana*.
Judith had the forty-plus class of students standing around me. It
was a whole new world for me. I had never been in a class where
people stopped and looked at you. As she gave me instructions, I
had perspiration coming out of me horizontally.

Progressively in that two-hour class, my sense of knowing anything about yoga dissolved. I was humbled by the whole experience.
I felt like a little kid. It seemed everybody was at least two feet
taller than I was. After class, I went to Judith and said, "I don't

know anything. Do you have a beginner's class?" She said one was starting in fifteen minutes, and I decided to stay. I put so much energy into it that my legs were vibrating. I couldn't believe it. When I walked back to where I was staying, with every step on those hills in San Francisco, I was going, "Oh! Ow! Ouch!"

I realized I didn't know much about the body. I had been studying yoga philosophy and knew the basics of posture and breath. But the depth and mechanics Judith expressed and presented were so much greater than what I had even conceived of, that I decided I really needed to delve into the practice of Iyengar yoga intensely.

I was also studying other traditions to experience the full spectrum. In 1987, I studied with Pattabhi Jois in Santa Barbara and San Francisco. I met Desikachar that year. The Iyengar practice was something I really wanted to get into, because it was much clearer about alignment, which was most foundational. As I did more *vinyasa*, I realized if I didn't know how to do the pose there was a greater risk of injury.

Are you still aligned with the Iyengar tradition?

Not formally. About three years ago, I realized the philosophy I adhered to and the basic parts of my practice didn't align with Mr. Iyengar's philosophy and the way he practiced. I slowly developed out of the system, and last year I formally resigned my Iyengar certification. It was an honoring to Mr. Iyengar, because I was teaching philosophy and alignment in a way he wouldn't fully approve of. It was dishonorable and dishonest to continue to use his name for my teaching. And yet, there are so many things I teach and practice that are directly from him. He and his senior teachers have made the biggest impact on a technical level, and I will always honor that.

I teach technical alignment, which Mr. Iyengar emphasizes, but instead of giving a lot of little points of alignment, I use bigger instructions, broader strokes. I use more instructions about how to work with the subtle body, the energetic body, which I call energy loops and spirals. I call my method *Anusara* yoga.

What is Anusara yoga?

Anusara means to step into the current of divine will, to move with the flow of grace. *Anusara* is about opening to every part of ourselves and seeing every part as sacred, seeing everything as supreme consciousness. Instead of making a dualistic system by saying the body is just a casing for the spirit and we have to subjugate the body, or control the body, or discipline the body so we can penetrate to find the spirit, we see the body as beautiful, even though it's transitory. Our body is our laboratory.

You are supreme, and there is tremendous goodness and worthiness inside of you. Find the blessing in your limitations, instead of seeing them as a curse.

When did you begin the practice of yoga?

My interest in yoga started before I practiced formally. When I was eight, my mother read me stories about yogis in the Himalayas who had supernatural powers.

I started practicing yoga formally when I was thirteen. I got some hatha yoga books and started following the photographs and the descriptions. The first book was *Integral Hatha Yoga* with Swami Satchidananda. There wasn't much explanation as to how to do the poses. I would look at the photograph to imitate and end up crashing into my mother's furniture. My mother still has photographs of me trying to do headstand in the middle of the living room.

Your mother sounds like an interesting lady.

My mother is special. She gave me my first chemistry set when I was three.

The junior welding set at four.

It was weird. I got rocket ships in those first few years. She always encouraged me to do what was true to my heart. When I was into yoga and doing really weird things as a kid, even though she didn't fully understand it, she supported me and my sense of discovery and investigation.

She gave me boundaries, but she let me grow my feathers, so I could fly out of the nest. If you don't allow the baby bird to grow the feathers, then the cat will eat it. I went to work when I was fourteen sweeping the floor in a pizza parlor. I walked home at night. When I was sixteen, she gave me a bus ticket to travel halfway across the country to see the King Tut exhibit. I was encouraged to play the edge where it's scary and free, and it's going to make you think. You make mistakes, but you learn to accept your choices and use whatever arises for your own betterment.

When I was thirteen, I read the Mascaro translation of the *Bhagavad Gita* and it rang true. It was so beautiful, and the teachings were so powerfully profound. I found a philosophy I could base my life on. I joined the local Theosophical Society and became the librarian, because I was in the library all the time. I was the youngest member of the group. I began to hang out with meditation groups. I became the mascot of the local Sufis. They decided I was very peculiar even for those groups.

My classmates thought I was pretty strange. I was one of the most unusual students at my school, but everybody respected me. I was a funny, normal guy, but I had this yoga and mysticism side of me that they never really understood. At my high school awards banquet, I was awarded the title of "Most Likely to Astral Project in an English Class."

They wouldn't have given you the comical honor if they didn't care about you.

I'm glad I wasn't a social misfit. I could really connect to all the different cliques—party people, drug people, intellectuals, and athletes. I was popular, but different. That was hard in high school, because you don't want to feel different. But I stuck to my convictions because they meant so much to me. I was this mature little kid who was really into yoga. I had a burning to know about life.

At sixteen, I had another profound spiritual experience that created a major shift in my life. The Theosophical people and the Sufis had gotten together for a one-day meditation. We were silent except for chanting. From early morning until late afternoon we meditated—visualizing and using our inner vision to contact inner energy centers. The whole day was so powerful that by the time I left, I was so naturally stoned I was seeing light outside and inside. I felt totally vast, expanded, illuminated.

I walked out of the house where we had been meditating. It was a gorgeous summer day. Everything looked different. Everything was bright, colorful, alive, beautiful. When I got home, my mother was cooking a Porterhouse steak, which was one of the family favorites. That was the big meal on Saturday night. I walked in and said, "Mom, I decided I'm not going to eat meat anymore." She thought, "We'll take John to the psychologist on Monday. He'll be okay." I intuitively felt if I ate meat, I would lose the ethereal feeling and get dense. For about twenty years, my mother didn't believe me. Every major holiday she would ask me, "Do you want the turkey leg today?" "No, Mom. Still not eating meat." She eventually realized it wasn't a fad.

How did you connect with your teacher, Gurumayi Chidvilasananda?

In October 1989, I went to India to study with Iyengar in Pune.

Then I traveled around the country and got sick. I happened to be in Goa, and I really needed Western food, because my stomach couldn't handle the Indian spices anymore. I had heard of an *ashram* in Ganeshpuri, north of Bombay, which supposedly had very good Western food. I decided to go there, rest for a couple of weeks, and eat some good food.

I arrived at the Ganeshpuri *ashram* in late October. The first question I asked the welcoming host was "Where's the cafeteria?" She asked me if I had written to Gurumayi. I said, "No, I don't know who she is, but I am really in need of food." She probably thought I was a tourist coming through without interest in her teacher, but she still welcomed me. For the next three days, I proceeded to sleep, go to breakfast, practice yoga by myself, eat again, and sleep. I totally took advantage of the facilities.

I decided I really needed to tell the lady of the house that she had a great *ashram*, and I was very grateful. Someone said, "Gurumayi is sitting in the courtyard this afternoon." There was a *darshan* line, so I stood in line and as I approached Gurumayi, I noticed there was a lot of *prana*, or dense energy, in the atmosphere. By the time I got right up to her, the *prana* was so thick that when she posed her first question, "Where have you been traveling in India?," her mouth moved but the words seemed to come out in slow motion. They hit my ears so much slower than the movement of her mouth that it scared me. I was speechless. My mouth was open. My heart was racing. I had expected to make a perfunctory type of acknowledgment. Instead, I was witnessing something totally unnatural.

There was a Western swami sitting near her. He touched my shoulder and said, "She-said-where-have-you-been-tra-vel-ing-in-In-di-a?" Over-articulating, as if he didn't know whether I was deaf or dumb. I told him I understood English. I tried to compose myself, and said I had been to Pune. "With Iyengar?" she asked. She seemed to know the answer. I said, "Yes, I am an American yoga teacher, I am in India studying yoga, and I heard your *ashram* had good food, so I came." She laughed. And then I said, "I do advanced hatha yoga, and I would be glad to give you a demonstration." I caught myself and I thought, "*What* did you just say?" It was the stupidest thing I had ever said in my whole life. The biggest demonstration I had ever given was at the YMCA for twenty people.

She gave me this side glance and cat grin and said, "We'll arrange it." She turned her head away and the *darshan* was over. I fell down and bowed. I stumbled away, went back to the dorm, and splashed water on my face. There was dusk light coming through the window onto a little mirror over the sink. My eyes were lit up like cat eyes shining bright, and I was shaking.

I went to bed that night in a dorm room of about sixty bunks. About two-thirty in the morning, I had this dream where Gurumayi came and stood in front of me. Her form was crystal clear. She didn't say anything; she just stood there. I was lucid, but I recognized I was in a dream. My eyes popped open. I was scared to death thinking, "This lady's inside me! I'm out of here!" I got up and packed my bags. I counted my money, and I didn't have enough rupees to get to Bombay. I had to wait until the bank opened in the morning. I waited on the bank steps, and this guy came and put a sign up and said to me, "Bank closed. Holiday."

In frustration, I went back to my favorite hangout—the cafeteria. A woman came over to me and asked, "Are you John Friend?" I said, "Yes." She said, "For as long as you are here, you are to teach the hatha yoga teachers." "But I'm leaving as soon as I can get money," I told her. "Well, Gurumayi wants you to teach the teachers," she replied. For some reason I said, "Okay. What time?" She said, "Four in the morning."

I taught a class and another class. Each day, I was looking to see if I could get to the bank. For four days the bank was closed. I was caught in this routine, and people were being super nice. Then I got this call [*phone rings*] saying that tomorrow at seven in the morning I was to give a hatha yoga demonstration in the courtyard for the entire *ashram* and Gurumayi. The *ashram* population was about a thousand people. I put the phone down and was afraid I would have a heart attack.

The phone ringing is a nice element of synchronicity.

Isn't that great? That's the way it works with this story.

You might need to get that. It's probably Gurumayi. Stranger things have happened.

Exactly.

I figured I had to do the most advanced demonstration of my life. I had to do the most incredible backbends, forward bends, twists, inversions, and hand balances. I had to be totally warmed up before I went out on stage. I got up at four o'clock the next morning to start practicing in the dark between the bunk beds in the men's dorm. One posture that I was worried about is called *durvasana*, where you put one leg behind your head and stand up on the other leg. It's a striking pose. I had done it before, but this time as I was bending the knee and bending forward to come out of the pose, I lost my balance. I couldn't get my foot out from behind my head fast enough. I stumbled, fell forward, and the top of my head hit the cement floor. I almost knocked myself out. I lay crumbled on the floor. All my fear came up. I was thinking, "This is going to be a catastrophe. I'm going to fall in front of a thousand people and humiliate myself. I can't do this."

I happened to look outside as the sun was rising over the village of Ganeshpuri, where the great saint Swami Bhagawan Nityananda lived and died. A few days before, I had been in the room where he had taken *mahasamadhi*, and I spontaneously sat down and started meditating. It was a simple room with a bed in it, but something about the room was so beautiful that I had cried.

As I lay on the floor that morning, I thought about Swami Nityananda, and I called out to him, really to God, for help. A cool breeze came in through the window, and immediately, I felt calm. My trembling stopped, and I felt composed. I had been comforted, and my prayer had been answered immediately. I thought, "I'm not even going to warm up anymore. I'm just going to have to give it to God, because I know I can't do it. I have to totally surrender."

I went out to the courtyard and stood by the stage. There was a chant going on in an adjacent temple. I looked at this little platform they had placed on the stone courtyard. The ground was not a level surface. The carpeted platform was slanted and elevated three feet. The first pose I was going to do was press into a handstand. I'm thinking, "There's no way. How am I going to balance? I can hardly do it on the floor. I'm going to be elevated on a table with carpet on an uneven surface." All my fears started to come back.

The night before the programming director had given me directions on how the program would go. He told me, "It's fifteen minutes. The MC will introduce you, the music will start, and you will start performing. You don't have to say anything. You can just do your performance." I went along with that.

Gurumayi came out of the temple when the chant was concluded. She sat in her chair in the courtyard, which then filled with people. It's showtime—cameras, music, MC. "Good morning, everyone. Today we're very happy to have with us a Texas hatha yogi who came here to eat the food." The whole crowd burst out laughing. I was embarrassed, but he said some honoring things and gave me a nice place. I got my cue, but I thought, "I can't just do this. I have to say something." I belted out, "I just want to thank everybody here," and spontaneously started giving this little speech. Gurumayi made a hand gesture to get me a microphone. Somebody grabbed a microphone and jumped to the stage. With mic in hand I said, "I came to eat the food, and yet you welcomed me because I was a visitor to your home. I am so grateful and moved by your open-heartedness that I want to give something back. My performance is my offering."

I put the mic down and stood on the stage. I put my hands in *namaste*, closed my eyes, and said a prayer. "Gurumayi, I need some serious help. If you are who they say you are, I need all of that." I bent over into *uttanasana*, put my hands on the stage, and started pressing up both legs into a handstand. It was like someone took a blanket, wrapped it around me, and lifted me up. I was upside down looking at my hands on the uneven carpeted stage. I stuck the handstand. I wasn't even trying. I opened my legs up and threw them into *padmasana* in a handstand. Perfect. For fifteen minutes, I flowed through this routine. I did poses I hadn't even planned to do. I felt totally supported. It was magic. I was detached, seeing this thing happen as if it was somebody else's body. I stopped, put my hands in *namaste*, and the crowd gave me a standing ovation. It was an incredible moment.

Spontaneously, I jumped off the stage and went over to Gurumayi and *pranamed*. I knew that was the first tangible grace I had ever experienced. I had read about grace in books for years and thought I understood the concept, but I believed grace was something someone might not experience in their lifetime. I experienced it there. It was very tangible. From then on I felt connected to her.

As soon as I got back to Texas, the phone started to ring, and I started getting more work. People invited me to teach, not only locally, but also nationally. I went from barely making it as a yoga teacher who contemplated going back to accounting, to becoming a successful yoga teacher.

How has your relationship with Gurumayi evolved?

We have become more psychically bonded. Our relationship is almost the same today in a lot of ways, even though I have been privileged to spend time with her. I see her every year. She often stays in her *ashram* in South Fallsburg, New York. I go there during the summer and teach.

Has the sense of awe diminished?

It's only increased. It's like seeing the vastness of the stars. It never ceases to amaze you. The more you know about astronomy, the more you are blown away. You start to realize how far away those stars are, how many there are, and how many galaxies there are. The more I get to know her, the more the mysteries and wonders increase. I am very much in awe. She is a real teacher and has taught me on a very physical, tangible level how to teach and how to be with people in my hatha yoga. I am very grateful, because I can feel how present she is in my life, and it's a gateway to something bigger.

Looking back, do you feel a sense of being called?

I don't know about being called, but I think we have certain things that are destined. Destiny is a result of our previous actions. We all have a certain *dharma.* In that way, one is called. We all have a natural current of talent and skill in our particular lifetime, and each of us has to find what that is. When you find it, there is a natural ease. You flow with it.

Yoga is not about control. For me, teaching has been the thing, but first and foremost I see myself as a student. That's the most important lesson—I am not ultimately in charge. I am not ultimately the authority. I am ultimately the student. Instead of me trying to control as the leader when I'm doing *pranayama* and *asana*, I feel like I am co-participating, co-dancing with so much greater energy. That brings me joy. There's a bigger ocean of consciousness that I am part of. This other part of the consciousness is the lead dancer and I am just following, but I am trying to dance with it as best I can. There are times in your practice when you hit that magical connection so deeply a beautiful ease arises, and both dancers dissolve into one dance.

Do you follow a particular religious tradition?

I am a student of comparative philosophy. I read Buddhism and practice some of the Buddhist tenants. My altar at home is Hindu-oriented. I love the Sufi tradition. By my bedside, I have the *New Testament*, the *Bhagavad Gita*, the *Tao Te Ching*, and the *Dhamma-pada*. Those are the things I read for inspiration. I find good in all of them.

I don't often suggest a student do it that way—to mix a lot of traditions. That's just the way my mind works. I like to check out a lot of different things and find a common denominator. It's not the easiest approach, because you can get confused when you take a lot of different roads. Many times, I will suggest that a student find what they are comfortable with and dive deeply into that. In America, we are more exposed to the Christian faith, so why not dive deeply into Christianity. I think that's honorable. But study. Don't be ignorant. Use your discernment, your discrimination, and study about the history. Find the roots, and respect the other cultures Christianity came out of. Those cultures are part of the Christian faith.

Isn't Jesus revered in parts of India?

Yes. In the northern part, they have historical documentation to say he visited certain places in India. Some scholars would question that, but I think it's very possible. The metaphors of the *Bible* have very similar references to previous scriptures that have come out of India.

What are the benefits of meditation?

Meditation helps you make practical decisions. You become much more intuitive. You might not know how a particular act or decision is going to affect you or anybody else, so ask yourself, "Is this the right thing to do for the higher good?" Something inside knows those currents, those ripples, way down and ahead. What is right is the natural, intuitive feeling of the heart.

The more you listen to your inner voice, the more you stay connected. I have to make choices. Is this choice going to bring fulfillment? Is it going to be in line with nature or is it going to be for the satisfaction of personal desires? Am I going to gratify a simple pleasure or am I going to go for something higher? The more I am connected, the more I know *this* decision, *this* choice, will be right.

My meditation practice connects me to the highest part of myself. I feel the natural goodness inside myself and inside others. There is a natural joy. Meditation is not this pinpointed focus where I block out everything around me or inside me. I am much more open to what is arising. I feel my thoughts and my body. By seeing what naturally arises inside, I see that these things are temporary, like the clouds passing in the sky. My witness consciousness is the unchanging blueness of the sky. Other parts of me are the clouds. They are quite beautiful, but transitory.

I gain insight and wisdom through meditation. Sometimes I get afraid or angry. That's natural. Those things come from the same place as peace, joy, and love. They all come from the same source, but the witness sees those things separately. The witness is much more steady and vast than the little clouds of emotion and thought that arise.

When I go into my heart, I feel love and experience vastness and illumination. The trick is to live that way when I open my eyes.

John Friend has been a serious playful student of yoga since 1973, starting at the age of thirteen. He has studied with a variety of hatha yoga teachers, most notably yoga master B.K.S. Iyengar. John is the founder of *Anusara* yoga, which is a unique hatha yoga style that combines universal principles of alignment with the art of inner body awareness and celebration of the heart. He is a regular contributor to *Yoga Journal* and has produced two highly acclaimed yoga videos, *Yoga: Alignment and Form* and *Yoga for Meditators.* Since 1989, he has been a student of Gurumayi Chidvilasananda.

ACKNOWLEDGMENTS

There are many important people I wish to acknowledge for their contribution to *Yogi Bare: Naked Truth from America's Leading Yoga Teachers*.

My family holds an important place in my life. I extend my special thanks to:

My wife, Mary Self, for enduring the late nights and for keeping the home fires burning.

My parents, Allen and Bonnie Self, for giving me roots and wings.

My aunt, Janice Mayes, for fostering a love of books.

A project of this magnitude requires the unique talents of many capable individuals.

Many thanks to Peaches Scribner, my editor; Lainie Marsh, my transcriptionist; Roger DeLiso, my typographer and graphic designer; Beverly Burge, my graphic artist; John Reiman, my proofreader; and Robert Wisehart, my Sanskrit consultant.

Other individuals have assisted me in bringing this project to fruition.

Thanks to Jan Campbell, Betty Larson, John Charping, Laura Tyree Hetzel, Diane Avice Du Buisson, and Zo Newell for helping to secure interviews and for your contributions to the Nashville yoga community.

Also, thanks to Leslie Bogart, Larry Rose, Joel Roman, Tim Schumacher, Joy Tillis, Ron Green, Alyse Markse, Paul Ringwelski, Liz Shields, Linda Corgozza, Carol Stall, Jonathan Pite, Sandy Joubert, Kathleen Mulcahy, Deborah Willoughby, Stephen Cope, and the staff at Kripalu Center.

The following people are acknowledged for a variety of reasons. The common denominator is they have always had my best interest at heart. That is the true measure of friendship.

My deepest thanks to Rev. Bill Stokes, Robert Guillot, Stephen and Anne Doster, Michael King, Sharon Pelton, Michael Dulaney, Janni Littlepage, Paul Dolman, Jeff Pennig, Donna Hilley, Darren Briggs, Alisa Graner, Patty Holmes, Michael Sandy, Mona Salinas, and Peter Scanlan.

Time is our most valuable resource. It is non-renewable. Once used, it cannot be replaced. To the reader, I am honored you have chosen to spend time with my book. I hope you consider the time well spent and are richer from the experience. I know I am richer from the time spent to share it with you.

Finally, the participants of *Yogi Bare*, through your commitment to yoga and choice of vocation, are among America's leading yoga teachers. I am privileged you were willing to share your vast knowledge and keen insights with me on a subject dear to my heart. Each of you has taught me through your words and actions. I offer my sincere appreciation and utmost thanks for your generous contributions and for sharing your heart. You have truly enriched my life.

Namaste.

Yoga Resources

Books

Beryl Bender Birch – *Power Yoga*
T.K.V. Desikachar – *The Heart of Yoga*
Donna Farhi – *The Breathing Book*
Lilias Folan – *Lilias, Yoga and You*
Lilias Folan – *Lilias, Yoga and Your Life*
Vyaas Houston – *Yoga Sutras Workbook*
B.K.S. Iyengar – *Light on Yoga*
B.K.S. Iyengar – *Light on Pranayama*
B.K.S. Iyengar – *Light on Yoga Sutras of Patanjali*
Gary Kraftsow – *Yoga for Wellness: Healing with the Timeless Teachings of Viniyoga*
Margaret and Martin Pierce – *Yoga for Your Life: A Practice Manual of Breath and Movement*
Erich Schiffmann – *Yoga, the Spirit and Practice of Moving into Stillness*
Paramahansa Yogananda – *Autobiography of a Yogi*

Video

Baron Baptiste – *Hot Yoga, Power Yoga for Beginners*
Baron Baptiste – *Hot Yoga, The Next Challenge*
Baron Baptiste – *Hot Yoga, The Ultimate Challenge*
Rama Berch – *Yoga for Your Back*
Alan Finger – *Yoga Zone Introduction to Yoga*
Alan Finger – *Yoga Zone Meditation*
Alan Finger – *Yoga Zone Pregnancy*
Lilias Folan – *Lilias! Yoga for Better Health*
Lilias Folan – *Lilias! Yoga Workout Series for Beginners*
Lilias Folan – *Energize with Yoga*
Lilias Folan – *Lilias, Alive with Yoga, Vol. 1*
Lilias Folan – *Lilias, Alive with Yoga, Vol. 2*
Richard Freeman – *Yoga with Richard Freeman*
Richard Freeman – *Yoga for Breathing and Relaxation*
John Friend – *Yoga Alignment and Form*
John Friend – *Yoga for Meditators*
Bryan Kest – *Power Yoga, Energize*
Bryan Kest – *Power Yoga, Tone*
Bryan Kest – *Power Yoga, Sweat*

Sandra Summerfied Kozak – *Basic Backcare*
K. Pattabhi Jois – *Ashtanga Yoga with K. Pattabhi Jois, First Series*
K. Pattabhi Jois – *Ashtanga Yoga with K. Pattabhi Jois, Second Series*
Erich Schiffmann – *Yoga, Mind and Spirit with Ali McGraw*
Rod Stryker – *New Yoga with Kathy Smith*
Rod Stryker – *New Yoga Basics with Kathy Smith*
Rod Stryker – *New Yoga Challenge with Kathy Smith*
Patricia Walden – *Yoga Journal's Practice for Beginners*
Patricia Walden – *Yoga Journal's Practice for Flexibility*
Patricia Walden & Rodney Yee – *Yoga Journal's Practice for Relaxation*
Rodney Yee – *Living Yoga's A.M. Yoga for Beginners*
Rodney Yee – *Yoga Journal's Practice for Strength*
Rodney Yee – *Yoga Journal's Practice for Energy*
Rodney Yee – *Yoga Journal's Practice for Meditation*
Rodney Yee – *Yoga Journal's Yoga Remedies for Natural Healing*

AUDIO

Thom and Beryl Bender Birch – *Power Yoga, Beginner*
Thom and Beryl Bender Birch – *Power Yoga, Intermediate*
Lilias Folan – *Lilias, Yoga for Beginning Student*
Lilias Folan – *Lilias, Yoga for Advanced Student*
Lilias Folan – *Rest, Relax & Sleep*
Gabriel Halpern – *Anger and the Warrior Within* (Dharma Talk)
Gabriel Halpern – *East Meets West* (Dharma Talk)
Gabriel Halpern – *Myth, Art, Creativity and the Elder* (Dharma Talk)
Gabriel Halpern – *The Geezer at the Crossroads* (Dharma Talk)
Gabriel Halpern – *The Guru's Shadow* (Dharma Talk)
Vyaas Houston – *Sanskrit by Cassette, Intro*
Vyaas Houston – *Sanskrit by Cassette, Part I*
Vyaas Houston – *Sanskrit by Cassette, Part II*
Vyaas Houston – *Sanskrit by Cassette, Part I & II*
Vyaas Houston with Mark Kelso – *Songs to Shiva*
Sandra Summerfield Kozak – *Breath Sounds*
Sandra Summerfield Kozak – *Relaxation*
Julie Lawrence – *Yoga for Health and Relaxation*
Erich Schiffmann – *Yoga with Erich* (nineteen separate live yoga classes)
Rodney Yee – *The Art of Breath and Relaxation*

GLOSSARY

Advaita Vedanta: non-dualistic school of Vedantic philosophy associated with Shankaracharya; the tradition of monism, which maintains that everything in the universe is ultimately One (Brahman)

ahimsa: non-injury, non-violence

ananda: bliss; joy

Anava-upaya: (1) "non-identification with the ego"; restraint of separation from the awareness of unity with God, (2) the technique of matching the level of practice to the student's individual needs (*see* viniyoga)

Anusara: "divine grace"; to be in the flow, or flowing with grace; to go with the flow of Divine Love

aparigraha: non-covetousness

asana: comfortable position; a bodily pose or posture

ashtanga: (astanga) "eight-limbs"; the eight aspects of yoga as taught by Patanjali in the *Yoga Sutras*: yama (restraints), niyama (observances), asana (postures), pranayama (breath control), pratyahara (internalization of the senses), dharana (concentration) which leads to the next step, dhyana (meditation) which leads to the last step, samadhi (absorption; the non-dual state of union or yoga)

ashtanga yoga: (astanga yoga) an intense system of hatha yoga introduced by K. Pattabhi Jois that synchronizes the breath with a progressive series of postures, producing intense internal heat (*see* tapas)

ashram: a yoga center or school; a hermitage or monastery

asteya: non-stealing

atman: the true Self or supreme soul, as distinguished from the consciousness or ego ayurveda: "Scripture of Life"; text and ancient Indian science of medicine

Baba Hari Dass: (1923–) A contemporary silent monk in Santa Cruz, California. In order to help quite the mind, he has not spoken since 1952, but instead writes on a small chalkboard. Author of *Ashtanga Yoga Primer* (1981) and *Silence Speaks from the Chalkboard of Baba Hari Dass* (1997).

Baba, Meher: *see* Meher Baba

bandha: to bind or lock; any of several muscular contractions, similar to mudras used to retain breath or prana within a given area of the body

Bhagavad Gita: "Song of God"; Hindu scripture detailing Lord Krishna's teachings on yoga to the Pandava warrior prince, Arjuna

Bhagawan Nityananda, Swami: *see* Swami Bhagawan Nityananda

bhakti yoga: "union through devotion"; the yoga of devotion to God, suggested by the niyama, ishwara pranidhana, and taught by Krishna in the *Bhagavad Gita*

Bharati: *see* Swami Veda Bharati

B.K.S. Iyengar: *see* Iyengar, B.K.S.

Bose, Jagadis Chandra: (1858–1937) B.A. from Cambridge; Professor of physical science, Presidency College, Calcutta; 1915, established Bose Research Institute in Calcutta; noted for his study of electric waves, and for his experiments demonstrating the sensitivity and growth of plants

Brahma Sutras: Hindu religious text, also called the *Vedanta Sutras*; written by Badrayana (Vyasa)

brahmacharya: moderation in all things; purity in thought, word and deed; also celibacy

chakra: wheel, or vortex; any of the energy centers recognized in yoga physiology

chi: Chinese word for spirit, energy or force; (*see* prana)

Chidananda, Swami: *see* Swami Chidananda

Chidvilasananda, Swami: *see* Swami Chidvilasananda

chit: the principle of universal intelligence or consciousness

citta vritti nirodhah: "restraint of changes in consciousness"; the definition and goal of yoga, as given by Patanjali at the beginning of his *Yoga Sutras*

Dalai Lama: (1935–) H.H. Tenzin Gyatso, the 14th Dalai Lama; spiritual leader of Tibetan Buddhism and formerly ruler of the country; has lived in the West since 1959; prolific author and speaker; received Nobel Peace Prize in 1989 for his continued nonviolent opposition to Chinese rule in Tibet

darshan: vision; the experience of spiritual energy from a divine being, spiritual master, or holy image

Desikachar, T.K.V.: (1938–) son of T. Krishnamacharya and yoga teacher to J. Krishnamurti; since his father's passing in 1988, he has been the leading proponent of viniyoga

Devanagari: "divine script"; the written form of the Sanskrit language

Devi, Indra: (1899–) Russian-born American yoga teacher; wrote *Forever Young, Forever Healthy* and *Yoga for Americans*; currently teaching in Argentina and preparing for her centennial birthday in 1999

Dhammapada: "Path of Virtue"; an early Buddhist scripture, consisting of 423 verses

dharana: concentration

dharma: divine law; the law of being; defined broadly as the way of righteousness or "that which holds one's true nature"; to "dharma" means to act in accordance with divine law

dhyana: meditation

drsya: seeable; able to be learned or understood

durvasasana: "Durvasa's pose"; a one legged standing pose with the other leg folded behind one's head

eka pada sirsasana: "one foot to head pose"; a seated posture with one leg extended straight out on the floor and the other folded behind one's head

ekagrata: one-pointedness; concentrating on one thing at a time; a particular attitude of total mindfulness during asana which allows all eight limbs of yoga to be active in each pose

guru: teacher; a spiritual guide

guruji: beloved teacher

Gurumayi: *see* Swami Chidvilasananda

hatha: The two syllables "ha" and "tha" represent the blending of polar opposites: "ha" represents the yang-active-solar-masculine principle, while "tha" represents the yin-receptive-lunar- feminine.

hatha yoga: "union through balance"; the yoga of physical perfection, generally considered to be preparatory to raja yoga; emphasis is on the first four of the eight stages of Patanjali's ashtanga system, especially on asana, pranayama, and pratyahara

Hatha Yoga Pradipika: earliest intact book on hatha yoga written by Svatmarama

Indra Devi: *see* Devi, Indra

Ishta: Lord, God

Ishta-devata: one's chosen deity

Ishta-pranidhana: attentiveness to God

Ishvara: Lord, God, Supreme Being

Ishvara-khyati: knowledge of God

ishwara pranidhana: devotion to ones personal deity

Iyengar, B.K.S.: (1918–) contemporary hatha yoga master in Pune, India; author of *Light on Yoga* and *Light on Pranayama*; has had a profound influence on yoga in the West through his training and certification of a very large number of hatha yoga teachers

J. Krishnamurti: *see* Krishnamurti, J.

Jagadis Chandra Bose: *see* Bose, Jagadis Chandra

Jains: religious sect emphasizing ahimsa (non-violence)

Jois, K. Pattabhi: (1915–) contemporary Sanskrit scholar and yogi in Mysore, South India who introduced modern ashtanga yoga to the world; a disciple of T. Krishnamacharya

K. Pattabhi Jois: *see* Jois, K. Pattabhi

kaivalya: (kevala) liberation; freeing one's consciousness from the sense of ego

kaivalyapadah: "Path of Liberation"

kapala-bhati: "skull-shining"; a rapid abdominal breathing technique used to clear the sinuses

karma: action; often misused in the West in place of "phalam," literally the "fruit" or results of action

karma yoga: "union through action"; the yoga of selfless action, where one acts simply because it is the right thing to do, without any thought of personal gain or reward; taught by Krishna in the *Bhagavad Gita*

khyati: knowledge, fame

Kirpal Singh: *see* Sant Kirpal Singh

Krishnamacharya: *see* Krishnamacharya, Tirumalai

Krishnamacharya, Tirumalai: (1887–1988) synthesized a vast amount of religious and yoga knowledge; important for his influence on the work of B.K.S. Iyengar, K. Pattabhi Jois, and Indra Devi, each of whom had each studied with him in their early years

Krishnamurti, J.: (1895–1986) world-renowned religious philosopher and teacher; founded Krishnamurti Foundation of America in 1969; "I am only acting as a mirror to your life, in which you can see yourself as you are; then you can throw away the mirror; the mirror is not important."

kriya: an action of purification, either spiritual or physiological

kriya yoga: the "yoga of action" taught by Paramahansa Yogananda; techniques of breathing and meditaion designed to quiet body and mind, and make it possible to experience a direct awareness of God's presence in one's life

kriyavati: with, or in the midst of, action; a state (akin to ekagrata) wherein the practitioner flows effortlessly into each asana, even the most advanced postures

Kumbha Mela: According to the *Vishnu Purana*, an ancient Vedic text, Kumbha Mela is observed every twelve years when the sun enters the house of Aries, and Jupiter (Brhaspati) enters what is known as the kumbha, or pot. In 1998, Kumbha Mela was said to occur in Hardiwar, India, shortly after the festivals of Maya-pur Vrindavan.

kundalini: "coiled serpent"; the latent energy at the base of the spine (*see* shakti)

kundalini yoga: "coiled serpent" yoga; an intense form of hatha yoga that encompasses many yogic systems and techniques designed to strengthen the nervous system and balance the glandular system for increased health and vitality

Lahiri Mahasaya: (Lahiri Baba) (1828–1895) initiated by legendary guru (Babaji) in the Himalayas in 1861; introduced modern Kriya Yoga in India

maha samadhi: great samadhi; a yogi's final conscious exit from the body and merging with the absolute

Maharshi, Ramana: *see* Ramana Maharshi

Mahasaya, Lahiri: *see* Lahiri Mahasaya

mala: wreath, necklace; a string of prayer beads; rosary

mandala: a magic circle; graphic symbol or symbolic pattern, often divided into four parts

mantra: hymn, verse; sacred power words used for meditation

Meher Baba: (1894–1969) born Merwan Sheriar Irani in Pune, India; called the "Avatar for the Age"; maintained silence from 1925 until his death; "I have come not to teach but to awaken. Understand therefore that I lay down no precepts."

mendicant: a wandering monk who has taken a vow of poverty

mosque: Islamic temple

mudra: seal; any of a number of gestures or bandhas used to control the flow of prana

Muktananda, Swami: *see* Swami Muktananda

mula: root, base

mulabandha: root seal or root lock; a contraction of the anus sphincter muscles used to concentrate prana at the root chakra to awaken kundalini shakti

nadi: "river"; a current or channel of psychic energy or prana

namaste: a gesture of respect performed by placing both hands together and slightly bowing the head; an act of respect, acknowledging the divine presence within each of us

nathamuni: "magical sage"

neti: a kriya using salt water or cotton yarn to cleanse the nasal passages

neti neti: "not this, not that"; a phrase used to suggest the impossibility of describing the experience of samadhi

Nityananda, Swami: *see* Swami Bhagawan Nityananda

niyama: observances; continuation of the ethics begun in yama: saucha, samtosa, tapas, svadhyaya, ishwara pranidhana

Om: The most sacred mantra sounds like "home" without the "h." Its three sounds (a, u, m) proceed from the back of the throat, through the mid-palate, and end as a close-lipped nasal hum. They are said to represent the entire range of human speech. Om is also used in all of the same situations where the word "amen" (Arabic: amin) might be found, including at the beginning or end of a prayer or reading of scriptures, as an epithet for God, and as the affirmation "yes."

padmasana: "lotus pose"; a cross legged position with each foot placed on top of the opposite thigh, used for meditation

Paramahansa Yogananda: (1893–1952) founder, Self-Realization Fellowship in California, and author of *Autobiography of a Yogi*; entered maha samadhi March 7, 1952

parivrtta trikonasana: "rotated triangle pose"

parsvakonasana: "lateral angle pose"; an even deeper side bend than triangle pose

Patanjali: (circa 200 B.C.E.) noted Indian sage who studied and taught yoga, author of the *Yoga Sutras*

prana: breath, spirit, energy, air; life force or spiritual energy

pranam: a ritual gesture of respect performed by placing the hands together and slightly bowing the head; to some it means "my soul bows to your soul" (*see* namaste)

pranayama: "control of the life force"; yoga breathing practices

pratyahara: internalization of the senses

purusha: pure consciousness, spirit or soul; the Supreme Being; pure, unmanifested consciousness

raja: king, royal

raja yoga: royal path of meditation taught by Patanjali in his *Yoga Sutras*

Rama, Swami: *see* Swami Rama

Ramana Maharshi: (1879–1950) modern Indian saint, born Venkataraman in Tiruchuzhi, India; taught maha yoga for knowing the Self by meditating on the question, "Who am I?"

Rig Veda: oldest and most sacred of the scriptures of India

roshi: "old teacher"; the Zen Master of a monastery; abbot

sadhana: "direct way"; spiritual practice

Sadhana Pada: "chapter on spiritual practice"; 1st chapter of Patanjali's *Yoga Sutras*

sadhu: holy man, ascetic, yogi, sannyasin

samadhi: joining, absorption; the final stage of yoga where the meditator joins in consciousness with the object of meditation; a non-dual state of consciousness

Samkhya: one of the six classical schools of Indian philosophy; Patanjali followed this school

samtosa: contentment

sannyasi: renunciate; also: a member of the Brahmin caste, once considered to be the spiritual heads of society

sannyasin: one who has taken a vow of complete renunciation

Sanskrit: the classical language of ancient India

Sant Kirpal Singh: (1894–1974) Punjabi saint who dedicated his whole life to the ideal of unity: the brotherhood of man under the fatherhood of God

sat: existence, being, reality

satchidananda: existence, consciousness, bliss; the ultimate nature of each individual soul

Satchidananda, Swami: *see* Swami Satchidananda

sattva: illumination, purity; one of the three qualities (gunas) of nature, the others being tamas (inertia) and rajas (activity)

satyam: truthfulness

saucha: purity: physical, mental and spiritual

savasana: (svasana) "corpse pose"; a state of deep, conscious, relaxation

shakti: power, energy; the yin or feminine aspect of spiritual energy, as kundalini shakti rests at the root chakra

shaktipat: "descent of grace"; transmission of spiritual power (shakti) from guru to disciple; spiritual awakening

shanti: peace

shishya: disciple or neophyte

siddhasana: "the accomplished pose"; a cross-legged position for meditation

siddhis: accomplishment; psychic attainments or spiritual powers acquired through the practice of certain yoga techniques

Singh, Kirpal: *see* Sant Kirpal Singh

Sivananda, Swami: *see* Swami Sivananda

sloka: short verse, especially one of Buddhist scripture

Sufi: "man of wool"; a Muslim mystic; pertaining to Sufism, the mystical order of Islam; these mystics used to wear coarse wool garments

surya: sun

supta baddha konasana: "reclining bound angle pose"

sushumna: primary central nadi located within the spinal column, through which the kundalini energy is said to rise

sutra: thread; an aphorism, precept, or teaching; a book of aphorisms

svadhyaya: scriptural study

svaroopa: (svarupa) "true form"; one's true nature

swami: "one who knows himself"; title for a Hindu holy man, such as a sannyasin, monk, or (more recently) a nun, who has taken vows of renunciation and lives a life of devotion to God and service to humanity

Swami Bhagawan Nityananda: (?–1961) "everlasting bliss"; Siddha Yogi, born in Kerala, South India; established an ashram in Kanhangad; guru who sent Swami Muktananda to teach in the West

Swami Chidananda: (1916–) "one who is in the highest consciousness and bliss"; disciple of Swami Sivananda; current president of The Divine Light Society at the Sivananda Ashram, Rishikesh, India

Swami Chidvilasananda: (Gurumayi) (1955–) current leader of Siddha Yoga meditation in India and in the West; Swami Muktananda's successor

Swami Muktananda: (1908–1982) received shaktipat (spiritual initiation) from his Siddha Yoga guru, Bhagawan Nityananda in 1947; brought this meditation tradition to the West in 1970; prolific writer

Swami Rama: (1925–1966) studied at Oxford and in Tibet, and with Gandhi, Sri Aurobindo, and Tagore; author of several books describing traditional yoga teaching in terms of modern science and psychology; demonstrated many yoga states (e.g. samadhi and stopping the pumping action of his heart) while monitored electronically at the Menninger Foundation, Topeka, KS, during the late 1960s and early 1970s

Swami Satchidananda: (1914–) "one who is in a state of pure being, consciousness, and bliss"; disciple of Swami Sivananda; founder of the Integral Yoga Institute and Satchidananda Ashram-Yogaville, Virginia; author of several books; gave the invocation at Woodstock

Swami Sivananda: (1887–1963) medical doctor, author, and founder of Divine Life Society in Rishikesh, India; teacher to an entire generation of yoga masters

Swami Veda Bharati: (1933–) a.k.a. Dr. Usharbudh Arya; child prodigy born in Dehradun, India; lectured on the *Vedas* and *Upanishads* by age eleven; holds several degrees; author of many books and founder of The Meditation Center in Minneapolis, USA

Swami Venkatesananda: (1921–1982) South Indian disciple of Swami Sivananda; maintained the Sivananda School of Yoga in Johannesburg, South Africa

Swami Vishnu-devananda: (1927–1993) "bliss of the Lord Vishnu"; disciple of Swami Sivananda; founder, Sivananda Yoga Vedanta Centre in Montreal (1962); author of *The Complete Illustrated Book of Yoga* (1960); accomplished small airplane pilot

Swami Vivekananda: (1863–1902) India's first spiritual ambassador to the West; represented Indian religions at the World Parliament of Religions, Chicago, 1893; author of several books in English

tadasana: "mountain pose"; the basic standing pose

tantra: "to expand"; the two syllables represent "warp and woof," suggesting the masculine and feminine principles that interweave to create the fabric of the universe

Tantra: medieval Indian texts on yoga and religion

tantra yoga: yoga practices for the expansion of wisdom and the awakening of shakti

tantric: involving the ancient tantra system of spiritual beliefs and yoga practices

Tao Te Ching: cryptic 6th Century B.C.E. Chinese text by Lao Tzu ("old master") that poetically describes that which cannot be described

tapas: heat; a profuse detoxifying sweat, generated by certain physical or spiritual practices; also: austerity, asceticism, purification

Tirumalai Krishnamacharya: *see* Krishnamacharya, Tirumalai

T.K.V. Desikachar: *see* Desikachar, T.K.V.

trataka: (tratakam) gazing; a visual technique to improve vision and concentration

trikonasana: "triangle pose"

upa: near

Upanishads: philosophical texts at the end of the *Vedas* where a teacher instructs his students; from: upa (near) ni (down) sad (to sit), i.e. students sitting down by a Guru to receive instruction

upavistha konasana: "seated angle pose"

urdhva kukkutasana: "strutting cock pose"

uttanasana: "intense stretch pose"; a deep, forward-bending standing pose

vanaprastha: "forest dweller"; the third of the four idealized "stages of life" in Hindu society, where one gives over all his property to his heirs and retires to a forest hermitage; the other stages are: (1) brahmacharya, the celibate stage of youth; (2) grihastha, the married householder stage; and finally (4) sannyasin, the wandering stage of complete renunciation of even the hermitage

Veda Bharati, Swami: *see* Swami Veda Bharati

Vedantic: "end of the *Vedas*"; based on the *Upanishads*; pertaining to Vedanta, one of the six philosophical schools of India

Vedas: ancient sacred scriptures of the Hindus

Venkatesananda, Swami: *see* Swami Venkatesananda

viniyoga: yoga adapted to the needs of the individual; to achieve maximum value, the practices are continually readapted to meet the student's changing needs

vinyasa: breath-synchronized movement; a fast flowing, aerobic style of ashtanga hatha yoga

vinyasa krama: "step by step progression"; a repeating series of postures, designed to systematically unlock specific aspects of the body and mind

Vipassana: "insight"; a Buddhist system of mindfulness meditation

virasana: "heroic pose"; either of several kneeling positions

Vishnu-devananda, Swami: *see* Swami Vishnu-devananda

viveka: discrimination; able to distinguish the real (sat) from the unreal (asat)

viveka-khyati: discriminating knowledge

Vivekananda, Swami: *see* Swami Vivekananda

yama: restraints; ethical practice in thought, word, and deed: ahimsa, satyam, bramacharya, asteya, aparigraha

yoga: union with the Absolute; any program for the attainment of that union; the ability to focus the mind and to sustain that focus without distraction

Yogananda, Paramahansa: *see* Paramahansa Yogananda

yoga-nidra: "yogic sleep"; where the body is sleeping, but the mind is awake

yogi: one who practices the discipline of yoga; one who has achieved the aim of yoga

yogic: pertaining to the study or practice of yoga

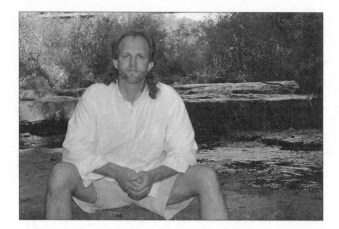

ABOUT THE AUTHOR

Philip Self is a music business executive specializing in film and TV. He received a Sociology degree from Louisiana Tech University and attended Candler School of Theology at Emory University. The avid yoga practitioner lives in Nashville with his wife and son. He can be reached at selfyoga@aol.com. His "Self Reflections" can be discovered at **www.cypressmoon.com**.

For additional information regarding the teachers interviewed in *Yogi Bare*, please contact:

Cypress Moon Press
P.O. Box 210925 • Nashville, TN 37221

T: 615-662-1867
F: 615-662-9385

e-mail: cypmoon@aol.com

www.cypressmoon.com